JULIA'S
MOTHER

JULIA'S MOTHER

Life Lessons in the Pediatric ER

WILLIAM BONADIO, M.D.

ST. MARTIN'S GRIFFIN ❧ NEW YORK

www.stmartins.com

Library of Congress Cataloging-in-Publication Data

Bonadio, William.
    Julia's mother: life lessons in the pediatric ER/ William Bonadio.
        p.   cm.
    ISBN 0-312-25251-X (hc)
    ISBN 0-312-27735-0 (pbk)
    1. Pediatric emergency services—Case studies. 2. Pediatric emergencies—Case studies. 3. Children—Wounds and injuries—Treatment—Case studies.
    I. Title.
    RJ370 .B66   2000
    618.92'0025—dc21   99-086893
                                                                  CIP

First St. Martin's Griffin Edition: April 2000

10 9 8 7 6 5 4 3 2 1

JULIA'S MOTHER

Julia

OCTOBER 15, 1998
THE EMERGENCY ROOM
CHILDREN'S HOSPITAL

3:00 A.M.

The ER winds down, like a wobbling top. The last patient is discharged home—at least for now. Still six more hours to go on this overnight shift. But for now the lights are dimmed low, as nurses brew more coffee and riffle through magazines to pass the time.

Will I get to rest a bit?

A cold chill always runs through me at about 3 A.M. It's the "night-watch" chill. We all get it. Drags on you, makes it difficult to finish an overnight shift. I can abort it—artificially— by taking coffee. A "caffeine push" is necessary at 3 A.M. when the ER stays busy, to trick the gears of your body through it; but you pay a price later on, because then you are nauseated for the next twenty-four hours. Or, the chill will resolve itself—

naturally—if I can get some sleep during a lull like this, to let my internal clock reset to a new day.

Sleep.

I move out of the ER arena to the adjoining physician on-call room. Go through an outer door—connected to a short passageway—then through an inner door. Now I am in. It's cold, and darkly quiet inside, with no hint of ventilation. Don't need much to furnish an on-call room—just a telephone, a pillow and blanket on a plastic-lined mattress.

You realize just how tired you are on an overnight shift after closing your eyes in a dark quiet room. It doesn't take long before weariness gives way to subtler shades of drifting. Everything is small, then big. I am joined to it, but not completely gone over yet. Then the boundaries of self begin to merge and fade, like drifting smoke from the lingering ash of a cigarette. . . .

And then it was my turn. It was early morning when the nurse came in to get me—I thought it was still night time, with the street so dark and quiet outside my hospital window. Saw her shadow above me rolling back the netting over the bed top, pushing down the side rail. She whispered, It's time to go, today you get your tonsils out. I obediently got upright and pulled the rope belt tight on my pajamas up around my chest, and put on my robe and woolen slippers. Didn't even think about being hungry or tired. Then there were two nurses, and they took both of my hands as we went down a hallway into an elevator. One of them said—Push the button with the 4 on it. We went up fast, and stopped.

The doors opened. It was quiet there—quiet and darker; the air smelled antiseptic. The floors were cold and hard, speckled like marble. We walked fast down another hallway; they held my hands tight going through swinging doors into a room with big people all around wearing masks and hats and white robes. I panicked when I couldn't see their faces, kicked hard to get away, but they grabbed me all over and I was floating and laid out flat on a high table. The big silver dish of bright light overhead burned my eyes. There were hands all over me now, holding my arms and legs and head, forcing me. Then a black cone came down over my face, hard and snug, and I couldn't breathe through the bitter hissing gas—I was choking, and it seemed I struggled out my last to get free. And then a man who was upside-down over me said, Don't worry just count to ten. There's a ringing in my ears, like a bell under water. I struggled out my last it seemed, sure that I was going far away alone and would never come back; then it all blurred, and the last of my strength was gone, so I gave in. I gave in. And the last thing I remember is how easy it was, to let go—how peaceful it felt, to finally pass over. . . .

Ringing . . . in my ears . . . like a bell—

"We need you out here—*now*."

The voice on the other end is . . . *emphatic* about this. I have to stay with it. Yet can't quite place where I am, or how I got here—

"What's wrong?" I ask.

"Motor vehicle accident. Child hit by a car."

Stark consciousness is jerked all the way back. Yet even with my eyes wide open, everything around me is still deep in black. I can't see my hands in front of my face—

"Are they here now?"

"No, not yet—three minutes out," the voice says.

"How bad?"

"It's serious—the paramedics sounded panicked over the radio. We only got part of their report."

"What time is it?"

"Just past seven. We need to get set up. *Now.*"

Now . . . it echoes like a rifle shot through my brain, as I grope to replace the phone on the receiver. Then pause in the motionless dark. *Just past seven.* It always takes a moment to accept that *yes I do have to get up, it's my shift, my watch* . . . then recruit the same automatic reflexes to fight back the temptation to doze again.

My neck and back are stiff, as if I've been down a while; I have to push my forty-three-year-old body through it, quickly, but in degrees: Sit up—shoes on—stand, straighten up, steady—shuffle forward—grope for the door handle—open the inner door. I reenter the dark passageway, the floor lit by flames of white light streaming in beneath the outer door. I hesitate to open it, anticipating the painful assault on my unprepared eyes—and then a searing white intensity beats upon my consciousness. . . .

There is only one thing I'm looking for—and I spot it, peripherally at first: The pattern made by the hectic pace of others, which indicates an impending crisis is coming—now—from somewhere.

7:11 A.M.

"They're here!"

The team rushes to their preassigned positions in the glaringly lit resuscitation room. Nurses, a respiratory therapist, several aides, and a pharmacist all scrambling at their posts to prepare—overhead lights are focused, machines whir into calibration, the cardiac monitor scintillates, IV pumps and tubes and fluids are readied.

The sliding glass doors open down the hall.

"Looks bad—they're moving fast!" someone calls out.

I know what that means. You get an early gauge on the prognosis of an injured child coming at you by the body language of the paramedics. I can see this crew far down the hall, quickly wheeling their load toward us like panicked pallbearers; shuffling sideways, stiffly hunched over their burden, looking down instead of straight ahead. I can hear the thud of their feet running. *This is going to be bad.* Now going past the empty waiting room area—and it's an all-out sprint. *Did something just get worse?* I can't tell, looking from this far away. The fluid bags and connecting tubes hanging above the stretcher clank in unison, like rigging on a ship's mast in a heavy wake.

"Should we call for a surgeon?" someone asks.

"Not just yet. Let's wait and see what we have here." You learn the hard way that too many hands can be just as ineffective as too few. There is time to call for their help, if we need it—

A last-second check—all the equipment is set up; everyone

is in position. Just a bit longer. . . . We stand in place, and wait to take it on. The resuscitation room is warped with tension. I can't feel myself inside the way I normally do. The rhythmic beep of the monitors on the stretcher rolling toward us intensifies. They've almost reached us now . . . then we grasp the baton, and run our heat with it.

"Everyone ready?"

I scan the faces surrounding me. There is no response to my rhetorical question, since no one knows quite what to expect. We've all been here before; yet each resuscitation is an unprecedented event. Which is why your chest feels tight and your hands shake. All you can do when this kind of reality comes at you from down the hallway is stand in, and take it on.

The paramedics rush headlong through the doorway. It's a young girl lying on the stretcher, wearing what was a white dress. We all strain to see, like wedding guests viewing the processional. Her clothes are sopped thick with blood. She has only one shoe on; the other foot is bare. I can see her left hand lying open at her side—the right is heavily wrapped in red-stained gauze. Surely I've felt tender hands and feet like these many many times before. But this is different—because there is no strength in her limbs, and because of the wet and dried blood staining everything.

The paramedics frantically steer the stretcher carrying the lifeless body up alongside the ER resuscitation table. They dock.

Do something.

"Make the transfer—let's go!"

Four sets of hands hastily reach in to grab a side of the undersheet support.

"One, two, three—lift!"

Now she has passed over to us.

Do something.

"Link her up!"

More hands reach in, to untangle the tubes and bags and wires, disconnect them from transport mode and reconnect them to our life-support system.

Do something.

Do something—now.

My first impression of her condition is the most important predictor: *Does she have any fight in her? Will the birth-cry force of life reassert itself?* But so far there's been no movement to her, none at all.

Despite the frenzy of it, her transfer to us was orderly. Each is doing his or her part, working together. My basic instinct is to jump at it—reach in both hands, take full control of the situation by doing everything myself. But to be most effective, the captain of the resuscitation team must stand apart, stay at the foot of the table—decipher the overall evolving pattern, direct the action and delegate to others.

A nurse with big shears is frantically cutting away the girl's clothing—her dress, tights, T-shirt, underwear drop wet to the floor. The skin beneath is so white, she's bled all the color out of it. No question we need more help—the calls go out: Surgeon, orthopedist, anesthesiologist, radiologist, intensivist— *to ER!*

The paramedics helplessly stand back against the wall to watch. One gives us report in a trembling voice: "Six-year-old girl—struck by a motor vehicle—crossing the street to school—"

He can barely keep up a full breath through the telling. I can only mind him with one ear, listening for any bit of information that might help to direct our attack, filtering out the tenor of his fearfulness as we continue to press on.

"At the scene she was unconscious, remained unresponsive during transport . . . shallow respirations—thready pulses and low blood pressure. Pupils fixed and dilated. Large laceration to the scalp, bleeding from ears and nose, distended abdomen. Major injury to the right hand. . . ."

Enough of this. I can see it all before me. I've heard enough to take over. We need to move on.

"The mother was notified by the police and is on her way here."

That sticks deep. And this is her argosy of pearls.

Do something.

The team needs to be given clear, strong direction. Measurements must be taken; priorities established; therapy administered. There's so much ground to make up here. I check the start time on the clock—

7:14 A.M.

"What are the vital signs?"

I snap out this first order as decisively as possible, to focus the efforts around me into some cohesion. So everyone knows exactly where the orders will be coming from. And to conceal my private misgivings: That there may already be an answer to the question which everyone here is surely asking themselves.

Numbers are the only comfort. They sanitize a medical emergency, allow it to be addressed objectively, dispassionately. I can treat *shock* more effectively than *this little girl's shock*. We will do our best for her if we don't feel for her, treat the problem instead of the person lying beneath our hands.

Her chances for survival hinge solely on the arithmetic, so I quickly take measure—heart rate, respiratory rate, blood pressure. I automatically tick it off in my head: Spontaneous movement—*none*; effort to breathe—*none*; palpable pulses—*none*; heartbeat—*none*. I've seen this null-pattern before—it's very, very bad. But there is a chance—if we can somehow find a way to recruit her languished strength to help us bring her back. It's happened before in this room. We must do it all for her now—rely on the science and medical protocols—then either it is in her, or it isn't.

One at the head of the table pumps oxygen to her shattered lungs through a breathing tube placed in the windpipe.

"Are we ventilating?" I ask.

"Both lungs, equally."

Another to the right of the table manually compresses her chest up and down, to circulate blood.

"Are there pulses with compressions?" I ask.

"Minimal—femoral pulses are barely palpable."

Several others are busy starting an IV.

"How many IVs are in?" I ask.

"Two. Two now. We're working on getting a third. What fluids do you want?"

This girl has lost a lot of blood. Even though her circulation is emptied, she's still bleeding from her mouth and nose and ears. There's no time to do a type and cross-match. She needs O-negative red cells—now.

I order a "round"—intravenous fluid and medications and a transfusion given in proper dosage and sequence, to fill her emptied circuit and charge it back into motion. The pharmacist quickly measures each, draws them up into syringes, passes them to the administering nurse; all are pushed through the IV with trembling hands. Continued ventilation and compressions. In a moment we will withhold support to gauge the effect. Either it is in her or it isn't.

"Hold resuscitation—"

We stop—everything is suspended for a moment—and peer at the monitors: There's no blip across the screen, no beeping sound; and still no movement to her.

"Continue resuscitation."

We begin again—ventilation, compressions; after a few minutes, I order another round given.

"Hold resuscitation."

We stop again—still no activity anywhere.

We start again, and repeat—this round, I order ten times the usual dose of adrenaline; a last-ditch effort to reach her stilled heart and jolt it into beating again. It is quickly pushed through the IV. After a few minutes, we hold to reassess. There is nothing, we are nowhere. So we start again.

As brave arms pull, dip and pull the beating oars, a silent black vapor overhead is sweeping the skies. And this young girl's mother is on her way here.

After three full rounds, it's time. For me to move up to the head of the bed. Just her and me negotiating this now. I retract the girl's eyelids; beneath it's lusterless, the eyes are marbled and vacant—raw, like uncut jewels. They move in blank unison like a play-doll's when the head is turned side to side. I focus a light beam into the corneal windows—her pupils are widely dilated, fixed in size—gaping, as if the tenant spirit was already released from within, had already passed. There's a perfume in her hair . . . beneath the coagulate her skull bone is crepitant, like a cracked eggshell.

The specter of death is here. It stalks the tall grasses on silent haunches, assured of its speed and strength. Yet we will persevere for the full interval— continue to press with what we know and what we have—apply external pressures and infuse corpuscular blood and artificial chemicals and bottled gases to try to push it back, to at least forestall the pronouncement. . . .

8:27 A.M.

We've been pressing hard to bring this little girl back now for over an hour. The first lab reports are just in; a crucial blood test confirms it—that her system has been shut down far too long. After receiving six full rounds of drugs, she shows no sign of any effort to breathe or heart to beat. Her blood pressure has plummeted to zero. The electrocardiogram traces the cold dark line of the horizon.

Individually—silently—collectively—we are resigned there will be no resuscitation here.

But when to cease, and let go? How long to keep at it? If we keep at it, could a miraculous thing perhaps take place? Can Divine Benevolence rectify Its mistake, and enable this young heart to pump out a line of warm red life again?

All of my knowledge and experience says *no*. Yet we are her only advocates. All are waiting, standing on the line. It's my turn to speak.

"Let's call it."

And with that, the formal pronouncement of death is made. Legally, it is the moment in time at which a licensed physician deems futile any further attempt at physiologic resuscitation. Metaphysically, it is a speck on a continuum; and we are merely porters.

Each of us peers deep into the blank monitor screen one last time, as if it might also tell *why*. The room is slurred, dimensionless for a moment. Then the certainty of science is relinquished. Surgeon, orthopedist, anesthesiologist, radiologist, intensivist; *clergy*. Now the individual parts of this case, which we tried to objectively isolate and deal with separately, are coalesced back into a whole.

The monitor scintillation effervesces away. Machines are switched off, disconnected, rolled back into the corner. It seems whenever we reach this point no one looks at each other. *Is that broken glass on the floor?* You think of the closest thing this could be to you—a neighbor kid, a niece, even your own daughter. . . .

Then the team disperses, and each privatizes their experience. Some have to leave. I know that some who leave will make a quick phone call home, just to check. Those staying begin to clean and restock the room, or do paperwork—any kind of directed activity that might make sense. Several nurses gently cleanse bloodstains from the reclining girl's still lovely face and ears and mouth and slender neck and matted hair with towels and a basin of warm water, then carefully dress her wounds with fresh gauze. The basin water is stained a rusty color. Rinsed down the sink drain. Soiled towels in the hamper. An aide gathers the pieces of wet torn clothing, and places them in a labeled plastic bag. A heavyset policeman uncomfortably paces the room, silently making notations.

I am drawn to examine the injuries more closely. *What was it that overcame her?* I need to know, perhaps the better for next time. She took a mean hit. Her skin is bled white and cold. Violaceous eyelids and lips. The abdomen bloated from massive internal hemorrhage. Her tender, unworked hand is severed at mid-palm—barely attached—the halved-ends of digit bones and fresh dots of scarlet marrow are visible on each side of the rent. Hand and eye injuries always bother me most. Her limp body devoid of its dolphin sparkle.

For the mother's sake, we must swathe these visible injuries in linen gauze before she views the body. Word is she has just arrived, and is in the "Quiet Room" down the hall.

"Shouldn't we go talk to her?" someone suggests.

"We" means *me*. What would I have to say? This weaver boy for the gods, clutching chilled red roses. How can I bring forth the telling of this? Make the necessary disclosure in the instant offered? The words, the manner of articulating them—will any of it come to me?

A final look back at the matter—her stillness is as a nightingale sleeping on its wings. She was only six years old when her hair was last braided, when she lost her teeth again.

As I begin to leave one task for the other, I realized that I didn't know this girl's name. How pitiful, that strangers can collide like this in a most remarkable interval for all involved, yet remain anonymous. She'll never know how hard I tried for her, let alone my name. I cut off her plastic ID wristband—*her name is Julia*—this is all the information I need to bring to the next task, which is to carry her name, bear it somewhere down the hall, and tell her mother.

What do I say to this mother? Giving this kind of devastating news is always the responsibility of the doctor-in-charge. Yet I'm not any more qualified to do it than is anyone else. In this business, there's no more difficult task than to leave a failed resuscitation to go tell a parent of their child's demise. It's a killing thing to do; it makes for more than one passing. There is never a kinder or more skillful way to do it—you have to feel your way through each encounter, hope that you can give them something of what they need.

But what do I say to this mother? I have to remind myself: *Don't think, just react.* Because they will drive the encounter. So you really can't prepare by trying to rehearse the "right" thing to say or do.

Go. I leave the ER arena for the Quiet Room. Pass down a

long hallway—it's a blur stretched out, like looking backward through a telescope. Round a corner—there it is; the door is closed. Will the words come? Will family or clergy be there for support? *Don't think, just react.* I've been here before—you feel like a nervous intruder going in; and an impostor when you finish and leave, because there is no greater truth than a mother advocating for her stricken child.

I knock, but can't feel the hard wood against my knuckles. What will I see inside? I carefully open the door—Julia's mother is alone there, standing in the corner with her back against the wall, her arms tightly crossed in front. Her face is flushed, her eyes so intensely focused on mine, her demeanor is vulnerable-pleading-defiant. *Walk toward her.* We are both lonely. Our eyes lock together—she sees inside me—the relentless fractional pause with no words between us tells all—

"Please don't tell me my baby's gone," is pled. The husky voice does not seem to emanate from her body. Now she is waiting, to hear if her name is called.

"I'm sorry. She did not make it."

This is all I can bring forth—I have nothing else, there is nothing left to give her. Like a deaf man singing an aria. Yet these words beat down on her with the concussive inevitability of hammer blows. She would not have heard any more. In the insupportable moment, time is everywhere—and her face passes through all of the ages. She turns hard away from the light and heat of it, covers herself with already sapless arms; and swoons low to the floor, deeply sobbing. Never heard anything so frighteningly mournful—like the howl of a majestic tree caught deep in the torrents, lamenting the torque that gripped its fresh season of flourishing leaves and pulled all down to ruin. . . .

9:00 A.M.

The overnight shift is ended. I pull the rope belt tight on my scrubs. I'm not ready to leave yet; it feels as if there is something unfinished, something left to be done. I want to linger, alone; but somewhere near by, not here.

Just before stepping outside, I recalled some advice given long ago to our medical school class by one of the professors, a retired heart surgeon named Dr. Fogarty: *"Always take time for yourself after the tragic cases; try to make some sense of them. Don't let them pass you by, or it will affect your practice later on. They are an important part of the journey. . . ."*

The medicinal airscent dissipates as I pass through the hospital exit. The sun is up again. I cross the sprinkled green of hospital frontage, then go down a short path to benches alongside the river. Overhead, the silent gulls skid down a gust on waxy wings.

This feels like a place where others have come before, looking for the same thing. I've been here before. You feel a bit older when you leave.

What do you do after a failed resuscitation, when a child dies on your watch like earlier this morning? You want to run out, but you can't. You want to scream at it—but you never do. Everyone else can cry, but not you. Instead, your insides go numb so you can continue to work. Doctors learn to mistrust their emotions, to push them down during a critical case, because they can interfere and block you from doing your job. Deny them—even long afterward—because there will always be others relying on you to intervene for them.

You never forget the deaths. Yet you go a long time numbed inside. Wonder why you can't feel for them, where your sympathies are. Then one day you see a cloud passing, or hear the wind in the trees, September birches—and your eyes mysteriously fail in their fullness. . . .

I looked across the way.

A group of schoolchildren passed by, walking in file two by two, holding hands like summerbirds. I swelled inside with joy to see them—admired their shining beauties, the surging energy, all the heroic potential . . . then was quietly despairing for them, these innocents paced into the uncertain future. . . .

You become an intimate of death, working ER. I've felt the mass of its sweep and pause in the room. Nudged it, pushed back at it with my own hands. Heard it lick the smear off its reddened jowls. Been sickened by the vulgar glut of its satiated leaving.

So I think I know a little about what it is to pass. Because I've been in the room with the perpetrator so many times. I know the children never pass alone—they take something with them, something important from their parents. The armature of infinity is relinquished; you can see it in the parents' eyes afterward—empty, wandering, perpetually vulnerable.

I saw it again this morning, with Julia's mother. Only one thing can cause such sorrowful grieving. Life is changed, after something you held to be truly yours is taken away, is gone; and you realize it can never be the same again. There's a cold spot on the sun, always a shadow as you go. You must start over, but with less; and can never fully believe in anything as being permanently yours. The concept of happiness is damaged, forever—like when the narcotics wear off, and the surgeon comes in to say they couldn't get all the cancer. . . .

I looked across the way.
City workers laid new pipe under the street. Old men with yellowed fingertips stood outside the tape and watched, remembering strong limbs. Their wives go to church on swollen ankles. Sometime soon an afternoon nap will merge into oblivion. . . .

I wondered if Julia's mother would ever be able to accommodate her daughter's death, and somehow be able to move on in her life. But then again, how could she? When all the mass of the seas and the light and heat from all the mirrored suns is insufficient barter to tip the scale back? A hungry pigeon will flock even to the illusion of a bread-giver . . . but where can she go, what can she ever do in this life after her loss suffered this morning?

• • •

It's time to go home. My scrubs are wrung through with sweat. No use changing clothes or even washing my face. Just go home. I don't feel hungry or tired, don't feel my legs walking out to the car. What I feel and what I think is disconnected—out of sync, on a delay.

I pull out of the hospital parking lot, onto the road winding through the medical complex. Trees, sky, clouds. Just like yesterday. Past the medical school campus. Those must be medical students sitting out front—some studying their books, some eating, others walking to class. It's always so jarring, just after the death of a child on my watch—to leave the ER and see strangers casually going about their usual business, living their lives. Eating talking laughing. *Don't they know what just happened?* I probably sat there too, a long time ago—studying my books, oblivious to the aftermath of a tragic case, unaware that some other disconnected doctor was driving by.

After a shift like this, you leave work and rush out ejected like a lit bullet. Try to estimate the toll it takes on you; like peeling back the leaves of an artichoke. And you begin to wonder where your life is going. Sometimes it's clear that something bigger than you is dictating the outcome; especially after contending with it and having nothing to show for all the effort. And your thoughts begin to wander in a dangerous direction, looking at the wisp of a span you're given in this life, and wondering if it's ever really worth it—if anything you do ever really makes a difference. . . .

"Take time, try to make sense of the tragic cases; they are an important part of the journey. . . ." Leaving the ER that day I had no idea there would be another encounter with Julia's mother, some months later—an unexpected one, which would permanently change my perspective—not only as a doctor, but also as a human being. . . .

After the Dissociation

WINTER OF 1977–1978
CADAVER LAB
STATE MEDICAL SCHOOL

O K, students—go ahead and uncover your cadavers," the anatomy professor instructed. A loud unison crackle filled the cold lab room, as the plastic tarps are retracted and folded and placed beneath the steel tables.

There it is. My cadaver. Lying on the gurney, stark naked. I recoil back a full step. *It's a—a "she"—* an elderly woman. Had to scan her first. The only way to tell is by the genitalia. Otherwise, there are no distinguishing features about her—like they'd all been smudged off. No hair—the dunk in the vat of formaldehyde in the basement had singed it all away. Her skin and breasts withered, the torso bloated. Everything a waxy, dull-tan color. Stiff and woody, like a mannequin.

I look away from her. I want to look back again. *Are the other students looking, or not?* After a moment of standing and waiting and not looking, I get up enough nerve; when it seems no one is looking at me, I look at her. Then I reach down to touch her hand—it is cold and stiff, feels artificial. The clear part of her eyes is thick and cloudy, lacquered. There's no expression on her face—nothing to tell of her final moments, whether she struggled or not. *What was her name? Where did she live and work? How did she die? I wonder what made her decide to donate herself to this purpose—it must have taken some courage to do it.*

Is this really a dead body? I keep looking at her, staring while trying to act as if I'm not staring. I expect her to move, to utter a word. So strange, to see no motion to any of it . . . unless I stare too long, and then my mind plays tricks on my senses—because every so often there seems to be just the slightest change in something physical about it. . . .

Formaldehyde. A medical student never forgets the greasy toxic odor of formaldehyde. It shadows you everywhere in cadaver lab during the first year of medical school. You take it home every night. Can't wash it out of clothing. Penetrates skin and hair, books. Must even coat the tongue, because you can't taste food all winter long.

All winter long. Cadaver lab means dissecting through a real dead body every day for six months, October to April of freshman year in medical school. Each lesson in the workbook guides you through a different body region—two weeks dissecting the abdomen, two weeks on the extremities, then the chest, then the head and neck regions. . . . Cutting through tissue, removing organs, holding them in your hands to study.

We all expected the anatomy curriculum to be intense. Especially after hearing about the two suicides in the prior year's class during Thanksgiving break. There's simply no way to prepare yourself for the experience beforehand, to somehow negotiate-down the dread prospect of confronting and touching and cutting through a human corpse. And no time during it to take a break and catch your breath, to pace yourself so you can reflect on what you are going through. Because—think of it—there's only one winter for a future doctor to memorize all the gross and microscopic structures of the entire body. Everything from head to toe, from superficial skin to the deepest internal organ, and all their interrelationships.

Each day of cadaver lab begins in the early morning winter dark, and ends in the early evening winter dark. Then hours of private book-study late into the night. Seven days a week. Days without seeing any meaningful sun—which is disorienting, and plays melancholy on your mood. In one way, it's like living through the longest winter of your life—with so much material to process and memorize and then regurgitate at test time in order to move along with the curriculum, to keep pace with the class. Yet in another way, it's like living through the shortest winter of your life—because the cold gray monotony of each day runs it all together into a blur.

It didn't take long to realize I would need a routine to get through it. A daily, rigid, unyielding schedule to save time and keep me at my studies. Everything else could wait until next spring—dating, doing my laundry, even calling my parents for money. I wasn't going to leave anything to chance—so I rented an apartment in the Walgreen's building just across the street from the medical school; and just before beginning anatomy I had the oil changed in my car, and pre-paid my rent and utilities for six months. . . .

My routine: I get up at 5:00 A.M. each morning, to the minute (didn't need to set the alarm clock after a few weeks). Know exactly how far to turn the hot and cold shower handles for just the right water temperature. Shave every other day. Before school, I eat breakfast—two English muffins with butter and grape jam, three cups of coffee—at Walgreen's, in booth #4 with the good lighting and wide tabletop so I can spread out my papers and books. Always served by the same waitress— Helen. After school, I eat supper—the fish sandwich with salad and French fries—at Walgreen's, in booth #4 with the good lighting and wide tabletop so I can spread out my papers and books. And drink coffee—lots of coffee. Then head over to the library (with a roll of quarters for the vending machines) to study late into the night.

Study. Repetition. Drilling yourself on the material over and over. Textbooks, atlases, lecture notes. At breakfast, lunch, dinner. On the way to and from school. At the library. In bed at night. I've underlined the pages of my books so many times they have ridges, feel textured like Braille.

Yet even with all the repetition, it's shocking to realize how quickly you forget. Whoever was in charge back then decided to name all the structures in impossible Greek and Latin terminology. Like the *supraoptic neurohypophyseal hypothalamic tract*—that could've been a whole semester right there. Or the nine metacarpal bones of the hand—*scaphoid, hamate, capitate, triquetrum, trapezoid, hamulus of the hamate, pisiform, trapezium, lunate.* And these are just the bones in the lower half of the palm. It's impossible to memorize it all "cold," just as is. You have to "warm up" the material, by inventing jingles and rhymes to help solidify your memory. For these nine hand bones I used: *Shakespeare Had Coined The Title Of Hamlet Prior To Lear.* Not a good choice—because at test time it took forever to recall which two plays were in the mnemonic; and then I accidentally wrote *hamulus of the Hamlet,* but still got full credit.

OK. Finished with the hand section. Memorized the blood vessels and nerves and ligaments and muscles and tendons and bones. Even the different parts of the fingernail. Passed the hand test. Then it was on to the heart. . . . And just two weeks later, after passing the heart test, a classmate asked me something about the nine hand bones. *Are there really nine?*—I couldn't remember anything about it. Drew a complete blank— as if I'd never come across the material before. Greek to me— literally. *How will I ever keep all of this straight in the future?* Yet there was no time to dwell on that insecurity, because we were already deep into the kidney section.

On the first day of cadaver lab, we received orientation from the chairman of the anatomy department:

"Today you begin cadaver dissection. I want to stress what a privilege it is, to learn anatomy on a real human cadaver. Because many medical schools don't have these resources—so their students have to learn from animal dissection. Dogs and cats. Which isn't nearly the same experience. The cadavers must always be treated with utmost respect. These aren't 'John Doe' bodies fished out of the river; many are the remains of well-respected citizens—doctors, nurses, teachers, clergy—who willed their bodies to science to help further your education. You are to conduct yourselves accordingly. OK, break up into groups of six, pick a dissection table to work at. Come up when I call your number."

Call your number? This is it. No way out now. Time to face the instinctive dread fear everyone has about confronting the mysterious presence of disease and death. *How will I react when they call me up to the refrigerator unit and open that steel door? What if I lose control, and disgrace myself in front of all the other students? If I freeze up under the pressure of cadaver lab does it mean I'm not cut out to be a doctor?* I didn't want to go, yet I couldn't wait to go. It helped to be going through it with all the other students.

A thick cold mist billows out from deep within the refrigerator crypt. Inside—a gurney resting on a track with wheels, supporting the outline of a human figure under a plastic tarp protruding up like a mummy.

"Go ahead—roll it out," the professor says.

We line up, three students on a side, and slowly slide the gurney out—each grasping a cold wet handle, like carrying a stretcher. *Is there anything moving beneath that tarp?* The air is thick in my chest. I keep my hands far out along the edge. Try to one-hand it—but fumble, almost dropping my end—and have to regrasp with both hands. I didn't expect it to be so heavy; later I learned it was because the bodies were submerged for weeks in a vat of formaldehyde in the basement, to soak the tissues through and prevent rotting. Like an oil-dipped railroad tie.

I have no idea what is lying there beneath that tarp, or how it will affect me. I'd never seen a real dead body, not like this. Sure, I'd been to family funerals; but a wake is different, it's under control, has set limits: The undertaker chaperones the proceedings; the body is contained in a coffin, sanitized almost beyond recognition with makeup and covered in new clothes. You don't have to get too close to Uncle Louis, don't have to touch. But cadaver lab is—is lawless—a naked corpse lying raw on the gurney; you standing over it—touching it—cutting it open, exposing the inside. Disrupting it. *Could the dissecting possibly let loose something terrible in the room?*

Cadaver dissection. Six nervous students in each group. "Body buddies." Working three on each side, rotating responsibilities. One is the "book," who reads the step-by-step instructions for dissection; the other two are "blades," who actually perform the dissection.

First lesson in the workbook: Dissect a large skin flap on the chest wall to expose the rib cage. The diagram shows how. Take a pen and make dash-marks along the skin. Then make a deep incision with the scalpel along the dashes through the skin down to the bone. Then use a scissors and forceps to dissect through the tissues beneath, to free up the skin flap and expose the ribs.

Scalpel, scissors, forceps. The most difficult thing about dissecting is getting the first cut started. Too many interfering thoughts. *Does a cadaver bleed? What if I cut wrong, or cut too hard and mutilate the tissues? Can I ruin something?* Cuts are forever in cadaver lab, they become a permanent archive of your work. I shuffle my instruments; then clumsily take up the scalpel blade, hold it this way and that over the skin; procrastinate making the first stroke; study the diagram again; then reposition myself over the cadaver so my hands can work in private. My fingers feel thick and awkward, disconnected—as if frostbitten, because they won't move with my brain telling them *do it, just do it.* I finally strike—with a shaky tenuous stroke that hardly leaves a mark. Have to go over it again and again to penetrate the leathered skin and deep layer of fat down to the rib cage. When I look out of the corner of my eye around the room, I see everyone else is nicking away at it, too. We all worked up to a full deep incision after nicking at it little by little down to the bone.

Beneath the skin you encounter a deep layer of fat. Insulation. A yellow, greasy, blubbery oil—like thickened kerosene. Oozing out after each scalpel cut into the field you are trying to dissect through. Handling and sponging up and discarding so much greasy cadaver fat is a potent diet pill, makes you think twice about eating that candy bar just before bedtime.

Beneath the fat layer are the internal organs. The first body cavity described in the workbook was the abdomen: Liver, kidneys, spleen, stomach, intestines, adrenal glands, pancreas; all the nerves and blood vessels. Identify them—carefully dissect them out, and remove them—then dissect through each organ to study its structure. Spongy, squishy tissue; slippery to hold and manipulate wearing wet rubber gloves. Pungent odors permeate throughout the lab room—bile, urine, stomach juice, dried blood, stool from digesting a last meal—all competing with the constant odor of formaldehyde. It's a surprise each time, to find the real organs are right where the atlas shows they should be; exciting, like a tourist following a map to discover a famous monument. The organs don't just hang there— each is wrapped by a thin clear sheet of sheer connective tissue (it looks like food wrap) which runs throughout the abdominal cavity from organ to organ, firmly securing each to each.

Each new stroke of the scalpel is a further tenuous step out onto the ice. With each new stroke you ponder whether going deeper might cause something impossible to happen, like a howling sound, or the floor to begin to pitch, or perhaps a snowy blizzard to engulf the inside of the lab room. Yet each bit of dissecting draws you further in, reveals more of the seamless design. Understanding the logic of the construction helps to remove the fear. And reinforces your confidence that there's a natural order to things. The most exciting discovery is the simplest—that you don't need any special insight or knowledge to understand the construction of the human body. Because everything about it mimics the everyday natural world. Geometric cell-patterns of elegant spirals, perfect circles, pyramids-cubes-lattices. Branching tree-like circuits of blood vessels and nerves and ducts. Fluids pass and flow and are exchanged and pumped according to the principles of gravity, magnetic charges, osmosis—the same forces that pull and swell the tides, and guide the silent drift of planets out among the stars. You can't avoid concluding: *What a brilliant piece of work.* Can't avoid asking: *Who made it?* Can't avoid wondering: *It seems so fragile, so susceptible to disruption—how does it all hang together, keep working, keep from breaking down long before it does? This splendid magnificent glorious ticking machine—what makes it stop?*

It's eerie, to look down and see your hands lost deep working inside a human body cavity. Exposing the internal mechanism to the light of day for the first time, like an archaeologist shining a torch on a cave wall filled with hieroglyphics. Once started on a given lesson, you are so focused on a particular area of the cadaver that it becomes impersonal, like working on a model. But at the end of each day, when you stand back to see the shredded remains of your cadaver growing thinner and more hollow from the dissections, there is a strong reverence that this was somebody once. Your cadaver becomes something significant to you—the artifact of your anatomy experience. And something personal—a quiet comforting presence; a companion, there to help you get through the winter ordeal of learning anatomy. Some of the students named their cadavers—"Homer," "Sadie," "Ezra." Some felt a real empathy for their cadaver lying naked on the cold steel slab—and dressed them in a stocking cap, and thick woolen socks.

Sometimes I step back and look at my cadaver, and wonder about her life: *How did it all turn out? If I could ask her, what would she say was the most important thing? Her biggest regret? Tell me—does any of it really matter, after it all passes?* Stepping back like that frees you for a moment from the hectic study-and-test world of medical school—and for that moment makes it all seem so trivial compared to an entire lifetime gone by.

Study and test. Each Friday the professors set all the cadavers out on the steel tables, and stick numbered pins in the different anatomic structures. Then we anxiously file around the room, get thirty seconds to identify each pinned structure and write the answer on a clipboard sheet. When the bell rings you move on to the next cadaver. You can tell which groups performed the most exemplary dissections by the number of pins used. Our cadaver always has an average number of pins. It could've been worse—they never put any pins in the cadaver from Group 3. "Can never use this one," the professor said. "What happened here? Did you guys use the wrong end of the scalpel?"

A loud bell rings overhead. "The pathologist is starting an autopsy in the morgue," the professor announces. "Let's go down to the basement to watch."

We quickly cover our cadavers with the tarps, and silently trudge chain-gang style down the hallway to the freight elevator. A steel crosshatched gate fronts the old lift; the only thing to do on the slow tense ride down the vertical tunnel is study the changing pattern of brick and mortar.

It takes three silent trips to transport everyone to the basement; then we herd into the cramped confinement of the morgue. Cement block walls like a bunker. No windows. A dingy checkerboard-tiled floor. *Does someone really work down here?* Recessed in one wall—another refrigerator unit. One of its steely doors is open; the crypt inside—empty.

There is a noise from behind a curtain, drawn in a semicircle around four table legs and two human legs in dark pants. Then a male voice emerges.

"Here already? Gather around. I'm just starting the autopsy."

The curtain is retracted by the pathologist, standing over the pillared lifeless body of an old man laid out supine on a steel slab table. Edged by gutters. With a shower hose at the top to rinse the blood. The deceased man's head is uncomfortably flexed forward by a thick wooden block placed behind it.

"This old gentleman died of a heart attack this morning while shoveling snow. I'm going to open the chest cavity to give you a look inside."

Open the chest cavity? We haven't gotten that far in the workbook—

After the initial shock wave of this confrontation passed, I felt—a pity for this deceased man and his predicament. Even though I didn't know anything about him or his life, it seemed he was at his most vulnerable, with no humanity to any of it. Just another case number, laid out naked on a cold steel table in the basement morgue, subjected to dissection by strangers beneath the undignified glare of a white-hot spotlight. . . .

There are surgical instruments set up on a tray, and an electronic device which resembles a carpenter's jigsaw. *Surely that thing isn't an autopsy tool?* I strain my neck and bend forward at the waist, lean in to get a good look—but keep my feet planted firmly in place so as to not be tempted any closer.

The pathologist focuses the overhead spotlight onto the subject's chest. Then he circles the table back and forth, quickly working the dissection with his hands, at times depressing a foot pedal on the floor to click-on an invisible recorder.

Click—"Patient number twenty-nine. White Caucasian

male. Aged seventy-four years. Acute myocardial infarction."—
Click.

This is all so strangely different from cadaver lab, such a big
step closer—because the deceased man had been alive just a
few hours before—speaking, eating, thinking. His facial expression (which shows struggle) is the one he died with. His
fresh red blood is being spilt with each maneuver. *The only
thing more fantastic than this is to be the doctor managing the
case at the time, to be there when they actually pass. . . .*

The pathologist procures a large razor of a scalpel, and
makes a deep confident Y-shaped incision, beginning at the
right shoulder, smoothly following the under-contour of the
collarbone across to the lower neck; then up along the other
collarbone to the left shoulder; then makes the stem of the Y
with an incision straight down the midline on the breastbone.

"So that's how it's done," one of the students whispers. "And
no dash marks."

He quickly dissects through the tissue planes beneath the
skin, then places metal retractors to hold back the flaps—which
exposes the flat white breastbone, and the ribs inserted into its
scalloped notches on both sides. Next he takes the jigsaw, and
places the blade at the lower end of the breastbone with the
teeth pointed toward the head. He activates the device, which
makes a loud buzzing sound throughout the hot cramped
room, and without hesitation cuts through the length of it,
bottom to top. Unzips it. *How could the front of a man's chest
come apart that easily?* The stench of burning flesh and bone
is nauseating. Yet I can't help but lean in closer, to see more.

Then he brandishes a chisel blade, and pries apart the cut

edges of the breastbone—just far enough to insert a steel device that resembles a vice; yet when he turns the crank it expands, to spread open the chest wall and hold it open. Which breaks most of the ribs. The kind of bone cracking you can feel deep in your own teeth.

The thoracic cavity is now widely exposed. *This must be the most intimate, deep, and secret of body spaces.* The ribbed interior resembles the hull of a great ship. It contains the heart. A real heart. The windpipe and lungs. The aorta, and the other great blood vessels. Terrific things, which were warm and humming just a few hours ago; now mysteriously stilled and silent.

The pathologist continues at his task of dissecting through the tissues, cutting away the pericardial sac surrounding the heart with a scissors. Dictating with each maneuver: *Click*— "The epicardial surface is smooth and glistening, the coronary arteries arise normally, are distributed normally, exhibit a right preponderance."—*Click.* He works a scalpel and scissors deep in the chest, but I can't see exactly where; all I can see is a surface of pooling blood, with more and more of it staining his gloves each time withdrawing his hands. Someone behind me whispers, "What's he doing now?" And someone else says, "Don't know—but he can't go any deeper—he must be cutting open the heart."

Click—"The myocardium is homogeneous, red-brown, and shows evidence of infarction of the anterior and left-lateral walls. The leaflets of the tricuspid and mitral valves show no unusual features. The pulmonary and aortic cusps are free of vegetations. The coverings come neatly together. The diameter of the aorta is uniform throughout, with no saccular or fusi-

form dilation. The inferior and superior vena cavae are pat-
ent."—*Click.*

Then he pauses, with both hands deep in the chest—seems
to be working to free up something—repositions his grip—
and then, from the very epicenter of the body, slowly extracts
the thick, red, round, globed, muted muscular pump from
within. All of a man's heart completely detached and removed.
The pathologist holds the cleft halves of it apart for us to see
directly inside—

"I've exposed the interior of the heart," he says. "Look here,
along the upper ventricular wall. Can anyone identify the problem area by looking at this tissue?"

No one dares to move, much less hazard a guess. I can barely
take a full breath. The group leans forward in unison, like a
school of fish turning; all eyes are fixed down on the work to
avoid contact with the pathologist, which might signal a willingness to answer his question.

"What would you expect to see after a heart attack?" he asks
impatiently. No one offered an answer. "We don't have all day.
How about you?" He points at Steve, the student standing next
to me.

"I guess if there's a blood clot in the artery, the tissue beyond
the blockage will be damaged—I think," Steve replies with a
shaky voice.

"Correct. Now look closely at this area right here. Do you
see the different color of the tissues?"

I needed a moment—had to stare hard under the bleached
glare of the white-hot spotlight, to see the slight gradation in
color—but *yes, OK, there it is*—a small pale spot, with a pink

blush of normal tissue surrounding it. The damaged area is about the size of a dime.

"This is the tissue damaged from a lack of blood flow. Does anyone know why infarction of this tissue caused the heart attack?"

No one responds.

"Well then I'll tell you. The nerves to the ventricular chambers run through here. When the blood supply is cut off, the nerves are damaged—and the heart muscle loses its signal to pump. We should be able to work backward from this damaged tissue to find the blood clot in the artery supplying it. This artery here."

Then he takes a very fine scalpel, and makes a crisp lengthwise incision in the coronary artery. Inside is a tiny purplish-blue clump of blood—poison-blue—which falls apart like moist sawdust when he picks at it with the probe. I lean my body as far as possible to see without falling over. Yet even my closest inspection doesn't help to clarify how this tiny misplaced nuisance—a blood clot, about the size of a pencil eraser—could have felled this huge tree.

I distinctly remember the April of that year—my freshman year in medical school. I received a passing grade in anatomy; the winter thawed, the springtime returned; and I kept pace with my classmates.

And yet I was disappointed afterward. In myself. Because I didn't allow the anatomy experience to change me in the way I hoped it would. After having reduced things so, I expected to become a "bigger" person—by gaining a deeper understanding of what was really important in this life. Hoped to rise above the petty trivialities of my rigid schedule throughout the remainder of my medical education. But I wasn't ready for the anatomy experience to do that for me; it seems I still worried about the minutiae of my daily existence—tests and grades and bell-curves, keeping pace with the others, grape jam on an English muffin in Walgreen's booth #4—until the day the dean handed me my diploma. And later came to regret that these preoccupations had allowed some potentially wonderful moments to slip by me, unappreciated.

It took many years to gain a real appreciation for that privileged glimpse deep inside the human body. And to realize the impact it had on shaping some of my most fundamental concepts about life, by revealing something of what it means *to be*. How? By a simple deduction. Because after seeing the vanquished corpses all lined up and thoroughly dissected, I had to accept that hearts and lungs and intestines are generic; and that the human body is, after all, only a splendid magnificent glorious ticking machine, which can be silenced forever in an instant. The vanquished corpses. It made me conclude that they'd been abandoned by an *essential vital* thing, an *intrinsic cardinal* thing, which can be transformed but not destroyed—which invigorates the body, flicks the engine switch to set it into motion, creates a history.

An essential vital thing. When my cadaver lady was infused by it during her life, she had a fingerprint; she was somebody's daughter, sister, wife, mother, grandmother. She moved in time; her heart raced with excitement and joy and fear; her brain anticipated, and considered—and eventually acquiesced;

her hands created and destroyed; her eyes gazed on beauty and on sadness, and glazed over during the final blurry moments of her existence. Then all of it was stilled and silent, a remnant; and what remained behind after the dissociation was simply the embezzled shuck, shed like locust skin.

What remained after the dissociation. . . . Coming up empty after dissecting a cadaver down to its ultimate physical essence caused an irrefutable, permanent split in my concept of man— into the two distinct realities of *corpus* and *spiritus*; and eventually caused me to conclude that the substance of each can be wounded, and require healing. . . .

Imperative

AUGUST 31, 1979
FIRST DAY ON THE WARDS
COUNTY HOSPITAL

*A*re those crickets making all that noise? Still pitch-black outside my apartment window. *What time is it?* I hear crickets, but no birdsong —seems the night hasn't turned yet. I've been turning, through most of it—shifting in bed, thinking about what's ahead today.

No use trying to sleep anymore. Not when my system is this charged up, jumpy inside. I can feel each heartbeat pulsating in my ears, like the red digits flashing on the alarm clock— 4:44 A.M. Better get up, there's a lot to do. Because today I cross one of those significant bridges—my first day on the hospital wards. As a "real" doctor: Wearing a white coat and beeper, carrying a black bag stuffed with shiny new instruments. Part of a real medical team making rounds, drawing blood, writing orders, standing at the bedside taking care of sick patients.

I sip a cup of hot black coffee in my quiet apartment, study the wisps of steam gusting about the surface, follow the sharpening degrees of my consciousness focusing. *Where's my check-list?* I washed the car yesterday, filled it with gas. Pressed my clothes last night. Even practiced tying my necktie. It took four tries just to get an even knot. They should make a clip-on tie for medical students with shaky hands to wear on their first day of ward duty.

Too nervous to sit anymore. I need to get going, get to the hospital, even though I'm three hours early and it's still dark outside. White coat on. One more sip of coffee—don't spill. Car keys. Ready to go. And for just a split second, I catch sight of something—dark—out of the corner of my eye; it shadows me as I walk out—startles me. I stop—it stops—I turn to look; it's my own reflection, staring back in the hall mirror. It cringes. *No—this is all wrong.* Looks ridiculous—distorted, like in a fun-house mirror. I'm puny; my white coat is huge. The black bag's as big as a suitcase. *Is this how I look going out?* What if someone on the street asks me about this get-up? What do I say? "No, I'm not really a doctor, not yet. Just a medical student. I've passed all the tests, so they let me wear this uni-form; now I'm on my way to the hospital to tag along and watch the real doctors work." Even though I earned the priv-ilege to take this next step, I feel . . . like an impostor this morn-ing. Because this uniform is an emblem, a trusted signal that the wearer has certain knowledge, certain capabilities. I have neither, can't meet that expectation.

I peel off the coat like it's on fire. Then fold it across my arm with the name tag-side down, draped over the black bag. And at the car, place them both neatly onto the back seat.

Better wait, and see how it feels once I'm at the hospital among the other students.

Headlights. Only a few all-night vans driving the dark open freeway at this early hour. There's State University. Hard to believe I spent four years there slugging my way through college pre-med—the proving ground—to gain acceptance into medical school. Going head-to-head with thousands of other college students from across the country who also wanted to be doctors. Competing at difficult science and math classes—biology, chemistry, physics, calculus; attending lectures all day, studying late into the night, an endless string of tests. Whether or not you made it into medical school depended solely on your pre-med grades—make the grade, or be eliminated.

It seems so long ago. Yet I recall every inch of pavement around that campus, because I walked it just about every night. Long private walks with my hood up, wondering if the book-effort and the classroom-sacrifice would pay off someday.

McAfee Hall looks the same. So many guys in that dorm wanted to be doctors. Yet only a handful made it into medical school—those with the drive to stick with the curriculum. The others followed their own curriculum—spending weekends drinking beer and shouting obscenities and causing minor vandalism. Someone always pulled the fire alarm late Saturday night. Weekend mornings they slept in late. The stories of these escapades were told and retold and routinely embellished in the cafeteria over dinner.

Although joining in on this stuff never appealed much to

me, I was tempted to go out with the others and let off steam after a full week of classes. But I didn't, because a night out represented five fewer hours of studying before a test. I had personal doubts each time I stayed in—*am I doing the right thing?* Spending weekends alone, confined to a wooden cubicle in a deserted library, memorizing my notes and book chapters, surrounded by the empty hum of the ventilation system— while everyone else went out on Fridays and Saturdays, and to the football games and to homecoming?

I'm not sure why I stayed with it. I remember the panic feeling inside, each time I thought about my future and came to the conclusion that there were no other options for me. Which is why I took the nocturnal walks around campus. Each time I'd ask myself: *Where is my life going? Will all this pay off someday?* There were never any definite answers; it was more like a sympathetic pep talk, a chance to say what I was going through, to tell myself how I felt about it.

At the end of each walk I'd remind myself *why* I was doing it—by recalling a conversation with our family doctor just before I began college pre-med. I asked him: *Was it worth it? Would you do it all over again?* And he said *yes,* without a doubt—because there is no other job in the world like being a doctor. No other work can make such a difference in other peoples' lives. Sometimes in a small way, sometimes in a big way. They trust you, depend on you in a crisis. They remember what you do for them. It's such a *privilege* to be allowed to practice medicine. . . .

I never forgot what he said. About the privilege. And even though I had no personal experience with watching a doctor at work, I understood exactly what he meant—that the opportunity to practice medicine could make all the difference in how you felt about what you did with your life. It always made me hungry to go back at it again. So I took it on faith—that the book-effort and the classroom-sacrifice of pre-med was to earn the privilege.

No more taking it on faith. Because today is my first day of hospital duty, and I'll be able to see and judge for myself.

First time through the gate of a doctors' parking lot. Like a new member of the club. Junior member. Better stay out of the way—park at the very far end along the fence. I can feel each step taken under the incandescent lamps lining the dark walkway to the sliding glass doorfront. The only person in sight is the janitor mopping the lobby. Like my father did for thirty-seven years at the elementary school. When I was growing up, my father would drive me past our town's auto factory during the summer heat and humidity, along the south wall where the tilt-glass windows opened onto the street, past the steam and the smell and terrible hell-noise crashing out; and he would always say the same thing: "That's where you end up when you don't go to college." On weekends he played drums in a band at the club to make extra money. One Saturday night I heard him come home late and put the drums away in the closet. He came into my room and woke me, sat on my bed. It was dark; I couldn't see him very well. The cloth on his suit was still cold from being outside, and I could smell whiskey or something. It scared me a little because he never drank liquor. He said he played that night for the doctors' Christmas party at the country club. Told me I should go to college to be a doctor when I grow up—that doctors are important, people respect them because they have an education and they do important work. Go to school, don't be a janitor, he said.

Two hours now before medical student orientation begins. I planned to get here early today, to walk the wards in private and get a sense of the place. Never been in a hospital at this early hour—it feels deserted. The lighting dimmed; there's no clinical buzz of daytime ward business. The only sound is my shoe-heel echoing off the polished terrazzo floor walking the hushed corridors. Who is manning the nurses' station? The doors to the patients' rooms are all open—deep dark silence inside, except for the red digital glow off the IV pumps and the bedside monitors. Throbbing red, like a bomb ticking down, waiting to explode. This must feel like so far away from home for them. What a lonely time to die in a lonely place like this—I wonder how it would even register?

There's a page overhead: "Attention—medical students report to the cafeteria for ward assignments."

We take our seats at the large oval conference table in the doctors' dining room, and pass around the assignment sheet. Which lists Dr. James Corrigan as my chief resident. *Chief resident. The boss.* It's intimidating to think of working with him—because I know absolutely nothing about patient care, and he's almost finished with his training.

As I made my way to the ward for orientation, I pondered the universal question of all first-day-on-the-job medical students: *What's expected of me?* We all asked it many times before starting ward duty—asked anyone who might know. *How do I act, where do I fit in?* And got the same answer each time: *Try your best to stay out of the way.* Because medical students don't perform any essential function on the team. They tag along at the back of the group, toil to make a spot for themselves. And observe. Things go better if you willingly accept the fact that the most you can aspire to during this earliest phase of clinical training is to be labeled as "useful"; which means eagerly completing menial tasks, consistently asking questions which show interest and initiative, and trying your best to stay out of the way.

Consistently asking questions. You walk a tightrope judging the best time to show how bright and eager you are. Have to pick your spots. You can ask questions—but not on the day after overnight call, when the team is dead tired; and not on weekend mornings, when the team wants to quickly finish rounds and go home; and not on Monday mornings before the team has had their coffee. It takes some finesse to judge the right time to ask questions. And a lot of self-control to keep quiet when it's the wrong time.

Dr. James Corrigan. Chief resident. Do I call him Jim, or Dr. Corrigan? I saw a polished and senior-looking doctor reviewing the clipboard roster of ward patients. That must be him. Neat tie. His white coat is perfectly pressed. Mine already looks like I rolled down a hill in it. What does it take to get that far? To be in charge of a sickward, able to handle anything thrown at you with such confidence?

Dr. James Corrigan. Dr. James Corrigan—

"Hello. Are you the chief, Dr. James Corrigan? I'm—" *I'm*

blank. He looks at me, waiting. By the time I recover, I've exhaled—am out of breath—and can't finish the last syllable of my name. Then I reach out a hand to shake his—and miss.

He takes us on a tour of the ward. Shows us the nurses' station, the procedure room, where they store all the equipment. Gives each of us a pamphlet on hospital policy and guidelines for etiquette and protocol.

"Each medical student will be assigned to follow one patient," he says. "I want you to actively participate in their management. Be advocates. Keep track of their progress; be alert to any changes or complications. Each morning and afternoon, the team makes walk rounds. I expect you to give a thorough presentation on your patient's progress. OK. Here are your assignments."

Medical student Claire gets "old" Mrs. Penny, a "frequent flier" here at County Hospital—seventy-three years old, wears a red silk caftan. Comes in about once a month—"Whenever my liver pills aren't working." Never anything really wrong. The nurses love her. Medical student Tony gets Mrs. Jones, a forty-five year old woman with a thyroid condition. And me? "Mr. Fredrick Ruckmeyer. A seventy-eight-year-old gentleman being evaluated for 'unexplained weight-loss.' He's in Room 444," Dr. Corrigan said.

Got it. *Mr. Ruckmeyer.* My first patient. I'm going to work really hard to take good care of him.

There is much to do before afternoon rounds. First thing—the most important thing—is to make a notecard. A four-by-six inch recipe card filled with the most vital medical information about your patient's case. Like a mini-chart. To carry in your pocket, and read from when presenting on rounds. To refer to when they fire questions at you in front of everyone—"What was the blood pressure this morning? What did the CAT scan show three days ago?" A nervous medical student can't count on memory to produce information during the pressure cooker of rounds. So you need a notecard. It's like riding with training wheels.

I hurry to the nurses' station, to review the details of Mr. Ruckmeyer's chart. Each section—page by page, line by line: Business and insurance information, historical data, physical exam data, day-by-day progress notes by physicians and nurses and therapists and consultants, lab and x-ray reports. . . . Copying the most important details of his case onto my notecard.

First pass through—*seven* cards. Way too many. The chief expects one, maybe two. He'll skip my turn presenting on rounds if I try to shuffle through seven cards. Yet everything listed on them seems to be important. Never worked through a chart before—what can I leave off? What if they ask me for some obscure piece of background information, and I don't have it? Then I'm standing there with nothing to say while everyone stares at me, waiting. Since he's my patient, I'm the one expected to know—

I shred the seven cards into a neat pile of squares, push it aside, and start over. Flip the pages in the chart back and forth, then back again. More and more abbreviations. Try coding in different colored inks. Lots of arrows. Second pass through— four and one-half cards. Still way too many.

Getting a bit panicky now, with only a few more hours until

rounds and no progress made. Let's try again—to take all this information and reduce it down to two, maybe three cards at most. In high gear now—coat off, the chart unfastened and all the pages scattered across the table. Got to eliminate something; let's concentrate on the hardcore medical facts and leave out all the personal background information—

"Can always spot a new medical student." There's a spinsterish nurse with thick ankles hovering over me like a bird of prey, watching me struggle. "By the shoulders. Tensed up to their ears. First day on the ward, right? Trying to get it all down on one notecard—right? You can keep trying. For now. But I'm going to take that chart—all put back together—to radiology with Mr. Ruckmeyer in two hours. Better finish up by then, or else."

Time to switch to writing with a fine-tipped pen. *Mr. Ruckmeyer: A seventy-eight-year-old male, hospitalized one week ago for "unexplained weight-loss." Admitted for "enteral feeding."* Enteral feeding? I looked up the term in the textbook; it means providing liquid meals by a tube placed through the nose down the esophagus into the stomach. Says here it's necessary for patients with impaired swallowing, like after the paralysis of a stroke. But nowhere does the chart mention that Mr. Ruckmeyer suffered a stroke, or has any other obvious medical condition interfering with normal swallowing and digestion. Yet during the month before admission he'd lost twenty-two pounds.

The book has a whole chapter on "Unexplained Weight-Loss." Gives a grocery list of possible causes. Cancer. Infection. Hyperthyroidism. Anemia. Inflammatory bowel disease. During his week in the hospital there were many specialists consulted, and many tests performed—blood tests, x-rays, scans of every major organ, scopes exploring every orifice. I abbreviate each of these, list them in a column on my card. And write "normal" after each one.

After seven days of forced tube-feeding, he regained four pounds. The day-by-day nurses notes reiterated: *Mr. Ruckmeyer is despondent, won't converse . . . refuses to eat or drink on his own . . . makes no effort to get up and about, refuses to watch TV.* This morning they wrote: *He awoke agitated and confused. It took several of us to calm him. . . .*

That's the last entry in the chart. A total of two and one-half notecards; written in very small script, with lots of arrows to direct me. A minor victory on day one of ward duty. It's the best I can do, short of putting it on microfilm.

Next step—to meet and examine Mr. Ruckmeyer in his room, 444, just down the hall. I put a blank card in my pocket to jot my findings on. Checked my black bag—everything's ready to go, the tools I need to use first are on top.

Room 444. I knock on the door. No answer. Is he sleeping? Or in the bathroom? I feel timid about intruding on his privacy. I'm just a medical student . . . but he should understand protocol at a teaching hospital, that we are all here to learn. I carefully open the door, only partway, and peer inside. There is the old man—lying on his back, deep under the covers. He is awake—his eyes are open . . . but looking away. Maybe he's hard of hearing. I need to note that on my card. There's the feeding tube taped to his nose, connected to the pump next to the bed.

Go. I walk in, and introduce myself. No response. His eyes— seem alert, but weak; distant, unfocused. Like a monument. Besides swallowing dry and hard one time, he didn't move or look at me. Is he angry? Did I disturb him?

"Dr. Corrigan assigned me to take care of you." This pronouncement didn't add any credibility to my cause, because he just lay there, his pale shrunken torso merged white-on-white with the smooth contour of the enshrouding sheets. His blank expressionless face makes no effort to turn and engage me.

Should I leave, or keep going? The chief didn't say what to do in this situation. I have to examine my patient before rounds, so I can make my presentation. Better unpack my bag, and see what happens.

"Let's start by taking your pulse." I carefully grasp his wrist between my thumb and index finger. Radial artery pulse. It's weak, thready. Weaker than even the tiny artery pulsing in my own nervous fingertip. I count out the beats for ten seconds— then multiply by six. Enter it on my card. His hands are rough and dry, the fingers twisted with thickly gnarled knuckles. Brittle fingernails, yellowed and deeply grooved. He has no grip.

"I can tell by your hands that you were a hard worker, sir."

His hand squeezes on mine—a little. Almost pulls on it. Barely. I looked at his face—his glazed eyes look back, focus on me for an instant; sharpen, like he's on the verge of saying something—

Then a cool draft of air combs the back of my neck, startles me—

"You'll have to finish your exam later." It's his nurse standing in the open doorway. "Mr. Ruckmeyer is due in radiology for more x-ray tests."

Better go eat lunch. They warn you early in your medical training—take any opportunity to eat, whenever it presents itself; whether hungry or not. Because you never know when you'll get another chance. And they warn that the only sure strategy for surviving a long-term of hospital cafeteria food is, simply, to avoid it. So you bring your own; or get something packaged, either by Mother Nature or by a reputable outside company. I got in line, and chose a cup of yogurt and a banana. There are two semi-agitated medical students in line ahead of me waiting to pay for their yogurt and banana, who seem to be comparing notes.

"What! You already made rounds this morning? Isn't the first time for everyone supposed to be this afternoon?"

"Supposed to be. But my chief decided to round twice today. It was terrible. I got sprayed-down in front of the whole team when it was my turn."

"Why? What went wrong?"

"This." The student with the blueberry yogurt produced eight notecards. "Dropped them when it was my turn. Couldn't get them back in order. The chief kept asking me for the blood pressure; but I got the numbers all mixed up. Then he went on and on about it being way too many cards—told me to bring a recipe box for rounds tomorrow. I would've had it down to a couple of cards by this afternoon. There goes my evaluation."

Better get back to the ward. I have to finish examining my patient before afternoon rounds. On the way there I can't resist the detour-pull of the newborn nursery, and a quick peek through the enchanted window at all the small warm bundles of pink smoothness lined up in their cribs. What a difference from the adult ward. No need for forced tube feeding here—the hungry ones exert the very pith of their lusty strength to obtain their objective. Each so eager to enter the fray: Crying, yawning, feeding, sleeping. All that optimism shining through the glass, like the earliest green shoots stirring through the moistened April earth.

Less than an hour now before afternoon rounds. And my first update to the team on Mr. Ruckmeyer. He must be back from x-ray because his chart is at the nurses' station. I reviewed my cards again, and silently rehearsed my upcoming presentation walking down the hall: *Mr. Ruckmeyer, a seventy-eight-year-old male admitted one week ago for a twenty-two-pound weight loss. . . .*

I knock on the door to Room 444. No answer. I open it, just far enough to see it's all dark inside. The air smells musty, like my grandpa's plaid winter coat. I look hard—almost can't find the outlined figure of an old man in wrinkled pajamas, lying on his side with his back to me, facing the window. The only sound is the barely audible whir of the feeding pump machinery.

"Excuse me, Mr. Ruckmeyer," I call in a hushed voice.

No response.

I cleared my throat again. "Mr. Ruckmeyer?" I whisper a bit louder.

No response. He should've heard me, if awake. Better not disturb him; hospital policy states that a medical student should never wake a sleeping patient to perform a routine exam. I'll come back and finish after rounds. At least I can tell the chief that I tried—twice.

The team gathers for rounds at the far end of the hall. Got my cards in hand. *Don't drop them. Keep them in order, follow the arrows.* Already decided I'm not asking any questions today; just going to watch from the back, see how it's done. Because it will take all my concentration just to present my patient to the team.

We begin the slow, methodical process of rounding, moving from door to door, each member of the team giving an update on their patient. Dr. Corrigan is all business. He listens to each presentation; sometimes nods at its sufficiency, sometimes asks a question or two, sometimes makes a teaching point. Jots notations on his clipboard roster. If there is something new to see, or something already noted which has changed, we all slowly pile into the patient's room and pack tightly about the three sides of the bed. The chief resident is always first in the room, and stands at the patient's right hand. Medical students are always the last in and the first out, like sweepers at the end of a parade.

For some of the elderly patients, sick and lonely and fading, this is the only bright spot in their day—the only point of physical contact, the only time anyone ever regards them, engages them, asks "How are you doing?" You can tell that some of the elderly ladies fixed up just before we came in, brushed their hair or put lipstick on. Their vulnerable eyes on alert, watching your every gesture; waiting. No easy way to finish and leave their room to get on with rounds when they want to talk—desperately want to talk, to leave a mark by telling you a little something about themselves, their lives.

But there's always more ward business to tend to—so after each presentation is completed, we move on.

About half way through rounds there's a page overhead: "Dr. Corrigan, please report to the nurses' station." He leaves us for about ten minutes. It breaks the tension of rounds, gives me a chance to turn away from the others and review my cards. *Keep them in order, follow the arrows.* My palms are getting sticky holding them.

When Dr. Corrigan returns, he asks, "Now, where were we?" and the team moves down the hall. Almost to my patient's room, 444. Hope I did the right thing by delaying my exam of Mr. Ruckmeyer, so as to not disturb his sleep. I can still update the team on today's vital facts: His calorie intake, consultants' opinions, new test results, the four-pound weight gain after seven days of forced tube-feeding. . . . My throat feels awfully dry. Nerves will force me to read the script verbatim off my cards at this point in my training; but hopefully, someday soon, I'll be able to present my patients from memory—

We rounded a corner. Then medical student Claire presents her patient, Mrs. Penny, in Room 443. "She keeps calling me *nurse,* and *dearie,*" Claire protested. I kept count—she used *three* cards to present to the team; that's half a card more than me. And no critical remarks from the chief.

We start to move again. I'm up next. *This is it, time to step forward—*

But Dr. Corrigan walks right past Room 444, and directly on to Room 445.

Wait a minute—there must be some mistake. Why did he skip my patient? No question about it; my cards show it's Room 444—the second door from the end. Even though all the doors look the same, I know Mr. Ruckmeyer is behind this particular one because I just saw him in there. Maybe it's urgent to discuss the patient in Room 445, and then we will return to 444.

I hurry to catch up with the team. *I must be up next.* Yet after finishing in Room 445, we move on to Room 446. *I have to say something about this, about missing my turn—I have to speak up—*

"Excuse me, Dr. Corrigan, I don't mean to interrupt, but what about my patient, Mr. Ruckmeyer: The seventy-eight-year-old gentleman admitted one week ago for an unexplained weight loss of twenty-two pounds who is receiving enteral tube feeding—back in Room 444?"

He glances over at me standing in the back, then down at his clipboard roster of patients, and casually replies—"Oh, you?" He mispronounces my last name, leaves off the last syllable like I did this morning when I blanked and then ran out of breath introducing myself. "Did I assign him to you? Well sir, it looks like we'll have to get you another patient."

"Why?"

"Because Mr. Ruckmeyer just died."

"*What?!*" I blurt out. There's a hot flush of panic rushing through me—panicked confusion—because I can't connect any literal meaning to his words. *His words?* All I know is that they are a threat to me. *Is this a joke? What did I do wrong? I just left him in there—did I miss something, and now my first patient is dead? Right behind that door?*

I've been cut loose from the mother ship—and am sinking fast. The other team members are staring at me—but I'm numb to it, already shocked past embarrassment. All I can do is inanely look down at the color-coded script and arrows on my cards, now illegible; then back up at the chief again—

"*Died?* When did this happen?" I ask.

"Probably a few hours ago. He was already cold when his nurse went in to give another feeding."

"*Already cold? But . . . what happened?*"

"Don't know. He probably just gave up. Let's move on."

Which is the last thing I heard, and could process, on my first day of ward rounds.

After rounds, I return to the nurses' station to review Mr. Ruckmeyer's chart. There is a serious-looking form stapled to the front—with the words "Death Certificate" printed across the top in large black letters. Filled out, and signed by Dr. James Corrigan. I scan it—at the bottom, under "Cause of Death," he's written—"*Lack of Imperative.*"

Lack of imperative? Never saw it mentioned as a possible diagnosis anywhere in the chart. I scour through the sections that I didn't include in my notecards. Under "Personal Information: Fredrick Ruckmeyer"—it states: *Current residence*—Springdale Nursing Home. *Prior Occupation*—farmer, for more than sixty years, retired; the family farm recently sold at auction. *Next of kin*—none; was married for fifty-two years; wife died from breast cancer six months ago; an only child, a son, drowned at age ten years. . . .

I shred my now-counterfeit notecards and toss them into the wastebasket. I need something tangible to fill this vacuum in my experience, something which is perhaps contained in Room 444. Again I confront the door; again, I'm hesitant to enter. I feel a compulsion to follow protocol, so I knock first; again, no answer. As the door closes behind me, the clinical buzz in the hallway drops out completely, and is replaced by another type of distortion.

The room inside is dim, motionless—the ventilation stifled and dense. Curtains are drawn across the window. The feeding pump and tube have been removed. There before me, laid out supine, is the old man—his mouth open, like in a scream. Just me and him on a warp. The inanimate shell lay blasted on the narrow bed, on sheets that would be laundered again and re-used in a different context. On the night stand is a pair of new hospital slippers wrapped in plastic, an empty water jug, a tray with some unused styrofoam cups, a tattered polaroid of a man and a woman and a boy on a farm. . . .

My ears are hot, and the strange metallic taste in my mouth won't clear with swallowing. *Just gave up? Is that all it takes?* I can only get so close, then have trouble drawing a full breath of this tainted air. I can't speak, even if speaking was the only way to gain my own salvation. Although the old man's life has expired, he's much more powerful now than I—much more powerful, because there's no confusion in him.

This apparition thickened the air. The specter of utter annihilation, of unreplenishable transformation, has a thrilling permanence to it unlike anything else I've ever encountered. I want to push it away . . . yet I want to get even closer. The reality contained in Room 444 has split off the screen. Because the syllables of this old man's life—the aspirations and longings and disappointments, the sufferings and achievements and failures, of one who had joined and mixed in the fray for that brief interval called a lifetime— they were all behind him now, echoed into the diminishing spiral of the annals of time. . . .

Imperative. I remember it was only much later in my career, after seeing this many more times and coming to understand it better, that I would think back on the context of the passing of Mr. Fredrick Ruckmeyer. They say most men die in earnest. But an old man is like a bundle of dried sticks—too many losses, and you disappear. He must have known his time had been. He must have been compelled on the day of his passing by a different kind of *imperative.* A force far greater than our medicine. A mysterious invisible power, working beyond the logic of science and numbers to coerce the outcome. The will to live can bring miraculous recovery when all hope seems lost—and, as with my first patient Mr. Fredrick Ruckmeyer, its relinquishing can nullify even the most effective proven cure for the most routine affliction.

I had to accept this—the compromise—that *imperative* was a given, that it had many faces, and would continue to mark the boundaries of my professional capabilities, either as an ally or foe.

Mysterious Urgings

SEPTEMBER 22, 1981
THE PEDIATRIC CLINIC
CHILDREN'S HOSPITAL

Seems I always make a wrong turn somewhere, no matter how many times I walk through this medical complex. It feels more like an airport—tunnels, lobbies, elevators, signs with arrows pointing in every direction. How does the public find their way around here? I still get lost, even though I've passed through this bustling place hundreds of times.

Cafeteria. Back in medical school I would veer left here, and follow the red carpet to County Hospital. Now, during my pediatric residency training, I veer right, and pass down the blue hallway every day to Children's Hospital.

Children's Hospital. Seems I made my decision to specialize in pediatrics by brilliant default. Backed into it—out of frustration, after seeing so many adults with medical problems due to their negligence, self-abuse, noncompliance—from smoking cigarettes, drinking alcohol, being overweight and out of shape, not taking their medication. I might have skipped a doctor's career altogether if the only thing to practicing medicine was taking care of sick adults.

A good choice for me, pediatrics. Although sometimes I need a reminder—like after a rough night on call, or when my pager just won't quit beeping. Then I go to the cafeteria, veer left, and walk the red carpet to County Hospital. Up to the fourth floor, over to the ENT cancer ward. I should mount a plaque there, in the TV lounge area, to commemorate the spot where I decided to specialize in pediatrics. It was during my last year of medical school. We managed an entire ward of adults who developed throat cancer after too many years of smoking tobacco, and required radical neck surgery to remove their voice box—had their malignant vocal cords and windpipe cut out. After which they were permanently mute, and had to breathe through a plastic tube—a tracheotomy—inserted into the front of their neck. On my first morning of duty, I asked the chief where all the patients were. "Been up and down the hall—the rooms are all empty," I said. And he told me to check in the TV lounge area. Which is where I found them—twenty-two speechless men, wearing pajamas and robes and plastic slippers, sitting silently watching a TV game show—smoking cigarettes through their trach-tubes.

Smoking cigarettes through their trach-tubes? Some wore a kerchief around their neck to conceal it in public; the cloth was always stained with brown tobacco spit. They coughed and wheezed a thick bloody mucous out the tube; had to cover the end of it with a finger in order to buzz out a few indecipherable words. One guy asked me if I had any matches. *Matches? Didn't you learn anything from all this?*

Whenever I go back to the ENT cancer ward for the re-minder, I vividly recall how difficult it was to work my hardest for them during that rotation.

Then I fast-forward a few months, to my first pediatric rotation at Children's. It was different. Toys scattered about the hallway, fingerpaint and crayon pictures taped to the doors and windows, popsicle treats and bright-colored pajamas and miniature chairs. The children are always blameless; their medical problems are never their fault. So your doctoring effort is focused on the more meaningful end of prevention, or reversing natural calamity. It's so much more satisfying to minister to the logic of their healthy young tissues, which have such great capacity to heal; and to enlist the aid of parents, who are so profoundly motivated to do whatever it takes to help their child get better.

Then I'm reminded. And can head back to work at Children's. Completely sure of my reasons; grateful for the contrast, the choice.

Friday afternoon—pediatric clinic is ending for the week. As I finish writing my last clinic note, tired, eager to leave for the weekend, one of the nurses—Roxanne—walks over and sits down.

"Mind if I run something by you?" she asks timidly.

"Go ahead."

"I'm not sure how booked-up you are with clinic patients. But there's a family—a mother and her son—the boy must be five years old now. They've been coming here the whole time and still don't have a regular clinic doctor. Someone who can really get to know them. So every time they come in they see a different resident, and mom has to start all over, re-explain his whole routine from the beginning—his medical problems, all his medications, what specialists he sees, everything. Which must be very frustrating for her—don't you agree?"

"Well, yes—I—"

Roxanne got up and stood over me, almost agitated. "And she can't ever seem to get anywhere with the boy, because there isn't one doctor in charge of everything. So I was just wondering, if you weren't full-up, maybe you could make room for them in your clinic schedule. The mom is so—*so earnest.* Her son is her life. She never complains, never misses an appointment, always gives him his medicine. I think it would help so much if she had someone to listen to her. You seem like a good listener."

What? A real compliment? My first, as a resident. How can I argue with that?

"Sure, I guess so. OK. Go ahead then, call her for an appointment—maybe in the next few weeks. What's the boy's name?"

"*Really??* Oh, wonderful. You're sure now? Thank you so much. She'll be so pleased. I bet I could contact her now, before the weekend. So she can come in early next week. Maybe even on Monday. Why not Monday afternoon? Afternoons are best for her, because she has to ride the Med Care bus to get here. Thank you so much."

"Whenever. What's the boy's name?"

"It's Clement. Clement Knight. But his mother calls him Clem."

• • •

I didn't think much about it until the following Monday, when I looked over my clinic schedule to see the name "Clem Knight" listed for the afternoon session. Still an hour to go before his appointment. Time for lunch in the doctor's cafeteria.

"Hey, is it true, what we heard?" one of the residents in line asked me.

"What's that?"

"We heard you got Clem."

"Got Clem?"

"You know—Clem Knight," another says. "Your new clinic patient. We heard you got him. Roxanne, right? She asked all of us, too. The senior residents warned us about it when we came on board."

"Guess I missed that part of the orientation," I mumbled.

"They call him 'tube boy'—because he's hooked up to so many machines. Just wait till you see his chart—"

Tube boy . . . wait till you see his chart. . . . After paying for my food, I sat quarantined in the corner to eat at an empty table. But lost my appetite, being too distracted with worrying about what I'd gotten myself into. So I hustled over to the medical records department, to review Clem's chart before clinic. I asked the records clerk to retrieve it for me—and she returned with five thick tomes of material.

"Got four other volumes on microfilm," she says. "Let me know if you want them too."

I reluctantly opened the cover of volume one. There's a form inside which all mothers fill out at each clinic visit—called

"Firsts"—on which they list the dates of their child's developmental milestones: "Held up head," "sat alone," "stood alone," "walked," "spoke words." Clem's form is blank, with only dash marks in the spaces. Signed at the bottom by Mrs. Knight. I re-check his birth date—*is he really a five-year-old?*

Which confirms my worst fear—this boy is severely handicapped, a tremendously complex patient with all kinds of difficult medical problems, all intertwined with each other. Pretzelled. And now I'm the one in charge of managing it. Here I've just begun my residency training, haven't caused any trouble so far, humbly accept the fact that I don't know anything yet, and already I'm in way over my head. . . .

Running late for clinic now. Got to hustle through as much of his record as possible. But where to begin with this huge volume of material? It's like reading through the Manhattan Yellow Pages. Better start with the "Clinic" section, since I'm most likely to encounter the same types of problems today.

I leafed through Clem's record; and by the time I gave up, had counted well over *100* clinic visits by the Knights—*in just five years!* Clem had been seen by just about every pediatric resident in the program at one time or another. But never the same doctor's signature twice. So there is no one in charge of his long-term care—no one to chart a long-term management plan. From time to time a particular resident would become inspired, and try to wean him from some aspect of his complex medical routine. Yet each attempt had failed, and by the next clinic visit he was right back where he started. Maybe Roxanne is right—maybe Clem could make progress if one person took charge and kept at it, took full responsibility for supervising these changes. Maybe.

I hear them before I see them. Big commotion—it takes most of the staff to clear the clinic hallway, to move the tables and chairs and equipment so Mrs. Knight can navigate Clem in his wide-back wheelchair—the one with the toy balloons tied in back, and the multicolored wheel spokes. Which also carries his life-support system: The ventilator machine, suction machine, cardiac monitor, three large diaper bags filled with his medicine and medical supplies. . . . Everyone says hello to them. Even the janitor mopping the floor knows Clem—who is sitting low somewhere in the midst of it, surrounded by the fortress of his life-support equipment armada. Five minutes early for their appointment.

"You don't need to rush in," one of the nurses advises. "It always takes them a while to get settled in the room."

After waiting twenty minutes, I walk in and introduce myself to Mrs. Knight. The back of the wheelchair is facing me. I can barely see the top of Clem's cowlick above the seat-back.

"So this is Clem. Roxanne the nurse told me a lot about him."

"We know Roxanne. Her little boy goes to our Special-Needs Clinic. He was in a bad car accident and has lots of problems. Same age as Clem."

"Oh, so *that's* why—"

I catch myself in time, correct myself mid-thought—"So *that's how* she knows you."

At first glance, Mrs. Knight seems to be soft-spoken and meek. Her voice trails off at the end of each sentence. A simple person—wearing baggy blue jeans, a wrinkled sweat-shirt, worn-through sneakers. No makeup or jewelry. Drab-colored mussed hair, in a tangle; the only glint of sparkle to it comes off the streaks of silvery gray. I can't guess her age very well—somewhere between thirty and fifty years old.

"Clem has quite a chart. I didn't get through it all yet. But I'll—"

"Don't matter. I can tell you what's going on. It's easier that way." She looks away when speaking, seems to avoid eye con-tact, almost as if ashamed of something.

Then she turns the wheelchair around to face me.

Oh my God—what? Is this really a little boy? I try not to stare, try to hide my startle at seeing the devastation up close, just a few feet away—the twisted withered limbs, the mis-shapen claw-hands, a grimaced face with saliva pooling and drooling from the mouth. *Is this really a little boy?* Roving, disconnected eyes like a shark—with no speculation or regard. The shrunken skull encasing a shrunken brain. The only sound he makes is the constant grinding of his teeth—like stones crunching under a heavy boot.

Never seen a child so completely shut out. Stuck in a bubble. He's shackled to so many tubes and wires and machines. . . . I try to control my reflex reaction—which is to flee the room, and get away to a safe place. It takes a long moment to accom-modate the distortion, this blur of a little boy reclining there. And to regain enough focus to speak again.

"I brought a new logbook to make notes in. Just for Clem's case. Do you keep a log at home?" I ask.

"Used to. Tried it for a while. But the writing tied up my hands too much. I need to keep them free, to suction out the trach-tube in his neck when he starts to choke on his mucous. *Like right now—*"

Clem is grimacing harder, struggling to move air—choking and gasping—his face is blue. *He's going to die right here.* Before I can stumble through a move to react, Mrs. Knight pulls on a rubber glove, grabs a long thin catheter tube, smoothly connects one end of it to the suction machine, disconnects Clem's trach from the ventilator, and gently suctions out a teaspoon of thick white mucous from deep within. After another minute, he is pink and moving air again.

"See what I mean? Don't take long for him to turn bad. One time he was choking and blue, the trach was so blocked up with mucous I couldn't get the catheter in—so I had to give him mouth-to-mouth, but through his trach."

Did she say mouth-to-mouth through his trach-tube? After all the commotion settles down, I said, "I brought Clem's chart so we can go through it."

"The other doctors said Clem probably got the meningitis germ from me when he was born. Do you think that's true?"

"Clem had meningitis?"

"When he was two months old. That's what started all his problems."

I began making notes. First section—"Past Medical History." "Let's start at the beginning. The record shows Clem was born at full term, after a normal pregnancy and delivery."

"Right. I had twins—the other was born stillbirth, strangled by the umbilical cord wrapped around its neck."

"But Clem did fine?"

"For two months. Then he got the meningitis infection. They said it was a bad germ for a newborn baby—strep-B. Do you think he got it from me?"

Didn't she just ask me that question? "I don't know for sure. But I've read that babies usually get that particular germ passing through the birth canal during delivery, and—"

Mrs. Knight had already moved on to the next issue. "The meningitis infection almost killed him. He was in ICU for three months; almost died every day for the first two weeks. But he made it. Miracle baby. When he was stable, they transferred him to the convalescent wing. He was there seven months recovering. Saw every specialist in this hospital. So now he's got all these medical problems."

She takes a worn piece of paper from her pocket, unfolds it, and hands it to me. There's writing on both sides. Different-colored inks, like it's been added to from time to time. I begin a new section in my logbook—"Current Medical Problems." Mrs. Knight sat patiently while I copied it—the list filled two pages. *Two full pages*—that's massive, by pediatric standards. The only thing I know for sure from looking at this list is that I have no experience with managing any of his problems—

"Clem's got brain damage from the meningitis," she says. "He's retarded. Blind and deaf. Can't breathe on his own—so the trach-tube is hooked up to the ventilator machine. It gives him breaths. I change the dials on it up or down every day depending on how he's doing. Another clinic doctor tried Clem breathing on his own once, but it didn't work."

"What's that tube under his shirt?"

"Clem can't swallow. Food goes right into his lungs and he gets pneumonia. So his surgeon made a hole through the skin over his stomach, and put in a feeding tube—I pump baby formula through it with a syringe to feed him. Sometimes I cut up fruit or a little chocolate and give it. Clem's got a bad stomach ulcer from the tip of the tube rubbing inside—when it acts up, he vomits blood. Then I have to take the tube out for a few days, to let it heal; and feed him with an eye-dropper so he doesn't get dehydrated."

I can barely keep up taking dictation. *Fruit, sometimes chocolate; stomach ulcer, has to feed him with an eyedropper for a few days when he vomits blood.* How's that possible? It must take her an hour just to get a few tablespoons of liquid in.

"Let's tackle his medication list next, Mrs. Knight."

She unpacks his supplies from the diaper bags. Suction catheters, bottles of saline, gauze pads, tape, rubber gloves. One, two, three . . . I counted thirteen freezer bags containing his medications. Each bag is labeled in dry-mark ink: "Seizure medicine," "ear medicine," "breathing medicine," etc. She lines them up on the table—opens them one by one, pulls out each brown bottle and describes the medication to me—what it's for, when it's given, how much to give, with or without food. She doesn't need to read the prescriptions. I list these under "Current Therapy." More like the index of a pharmacy textbook: Three medications for wheezing, an antacid for stomach ulcers, three for seizures (each requiring weekly testing to monitor his widely fluctuating blood levels), a daily antibiotic to prevent ear infections, a daily antibiotic to prevent kidney infections, valium to relax spastic limbs; two cardiac medications—Digoxin, to help damaged heart muscle to pump, and Lasix, a diuretic to prevent fluid buildup in the lungs; and a medication called Diamox.

"What's the Diamox for?" I ask.

"Clem's got water on the brain. It builds up because of scar tissue blockage in his neck. They put a shunt tube in his head to drain fluid past the blockage. His brain makes less fluid when he takes Diamox."

"You give all these medications every day?" I quickly did the calculation—"It looks like the only break you get is between 2 A.M. and 6 A.M. How do you remember it all? Do you set the alarm clock to get up in the middle of the night?"

"No. I'm so used to it by now. I always wake up when it's time."

After I enter all the information in this section of my log, I say, "Let's take a look at Clem."

Mrs. Knight unstraps him from the wheelchair and picks him up—his body is as stiff as a rusted springcoil. She lays him on the exam table. He gets even more rigid when he grimaces hard and arches his back. Every few minutes his eyes clench shut, his mouth opens wide—and he issues a noiseless cry, then goes into a spasm—arms and legs violently shaking for a few seconds. Then it stops.

Where to begin with all this? I'm afraid to handle him. What *can* I touch? Stay away from the tubes—trach-tube in the neck, feeding tube in the stomach, shunt tube in the head. I've never dealt with any *one* of these, let alone *three.* It would be a disaster if I accidentally snagged one, and pulled it out—because then he'd have to go straight to the operating room and have it replaced.

After another spasm-wave came and passed, I began my exam. He's so floppy—there's no muscle tone in his head and neck, no physical strength in him. He doesn't kick or reach. And that odor—from the sour stench of stomach acid mixed with digested formula coming out through the feeding tube. There's no enamel on his pegged, ground-down teeth; the gums are thick and overgrown. "His gums got thick from taking the seizure medicine," Mrs. Knight says.

So strange, to see a child with no sparkle, no new green pushing through. No purposeful movements. No smile, no regard or focus in the eyes. Withering, like the sibyl hanging in a cage. No curiosity, even with me shining the light. Curiosity—the most child-ish of things. Wouldn't he be learning his colors and numbers by now? The only regular sounds are his teeth grinding, and the wheezing and gurgling snorts coming through the trach-tube. And then there's that noiseless cry he makes just before a spasm.

How can I make any of this any better? He's so severely damaged. I can't imagine him being anything other than trapped in this bubble—attached to life-support machines, bedridden, wearing a diaper, only able to assert himself by struggling and grimacing a little more than usual to signal a need or a discomfort. His eyes will never meaningfully fix on the external world, his face unable to muster a social smile, his withered hands incapable of curiously manipulating a toy (although one of the diaper bags on his wheelchair is filled with them). He'll continue to make the constant gurgling sound through his trach-tube, which will require emergency suctioning to prevent him from suffocating on his own mucous. His spastic arms and legs will continue to shake and bow and wither more acutely. . . .

"Look at that!" Mrs. Knight says. "See him wrinkle up his forehead? I figured out he does that whenever he likes his doctor." Even though I didn't see what she was referring to, I noted it in my logbook.

After completing my exam, I sat across the table from Mrs. Knight. Time for us to discuss the plan. *Plan?* I have no idea where to begin. Clem's problems are so far beyond my junior level of experience. I'm sure she's got expectations—but where to begin? What should I say?

I silently review my notes again in the logbook. She sits quietly, waiting. Perhaps it would be best to let her tell me— so I ask, "Mrs. Knight, if we could work to make one thing better for Clem, what would you want it to be?"

"Well, the doctors who checked him before said he can't see or hear. But I think it's getting better. I'd like him tested again. Maybe he needs glasses and a hearing aid."

After clinic, I watched Mrs. Knight push Clem and his equipment out to the front entrance of the hospital, to wait for the Med Care bus to take them back home. She rummages through a diaper bag, looking for something. Waiting with the other mothers and children after their clinic appointments. The other mothers look at the Knights, then quickly look away. Some of the children keep looking until their mothers distract them. Some of the mothers look again, quickly, while trying to appear as if they aren't looking; I certainly know their thoughts. Mrs. Knight seems oblivious to it—to their sympathies for the squalor.

I spent the remainder of the afternoon reviewing Clem's chart, to fill in the other sections of my logbook. Under "Personal Information," I wrote that Mrs. Knight had three miscarriages prior to bearing Clem. There were no other children. She lived alone; there were no other caretakers to contact in case of an emergency, because both her parents were deceased, and she was divorced from Mr. Knight six months after Clem developed the meningitis.

I made the next entry in my logbook at 6 A.M. on Tuesday morning, the day after our first appointment:

MRS. KNIGHT PAGED ME AS I WAS DRIVING TO THE HOSPITAL:
CRYING, SAID SHE WAS JUST ABOUT TO TAKE CLEM TO THE
ER. SHE FELL ASLEEP AT 2 A.M., SO HE MISSED HIS OVER-
NIGHT DOSE OF DILANTIN. SHE WORRIED HE WOULD HAVE
CONVULSIONS ALL DAY, AND END UP IN THE ICU LIKE LAST
TIME. AFTER LOOKING IT UP IN THE TEXTBOOK, I REASSURED
HER THAT MISSING ONE DOSE OF DILANTIN SHOULDN'T
CAUSE MUCH OF A DROP IN THE BLOOD LEVEL-AND TO GIVE A
DOUBLE-DOSE THIS MORNING, TO CATCH UP.

I made logbook entries like that, page after page. Early on, when she called with a problem, I was afraid to handle it over the phone. So each time I instructed her to bring Clem to the hospital for direct evaluation, to meet me at the clinic and I'd squeeze him into the schedule. And she came, each time; packed everything, called the Med Care bus, rode the forty-seven miles to the hospital. If it was after-hours and the clinic was closed, I met them in the ER.

Most times it's been a false alarm. It's just Clem. After a while I learned about Clem, felt more comfortable with his patterns (none of which is described in any textbook) and became more liberal in recommending home therapy and monitoring. So that now, when his mother calls, I hear her out regarding his problem—let her tell it fully—and it's usually appropriate to say to her, "You know, we've seen him do this before, haven't we, Mrs. Knight?" And she always seems to be relieved to get the reassurance.

The change shows in the progression of my logged-in notes:

MOM CALLED IN A PANIC DURING CLEM'S BIRTHDAY PARTY—
HE'S WHEEZING, BREATHING HARDER, HIS LIPS TURNED BLUE.
I TOLD HER TO TURN UP HIS OXYGEN; FLUSH HIS TRACHEOTOMY
TUBE WITH SALINE SOLUTION, SUCTION IT OUT THOROUGHLY;
THEN GIVE THREE AEROSOL INHALATION TREATMENTS IN A
ROW; THEN GIVE THE STEROID MEDICATION FOR THE NEXT
FOUR DAYS. CALL BACK IF NOT IMPROVED BY MORNING—

And,

MOM CALLED-VERY UPSET-CLEM GOT SICK AT THE ZOO, ISN'T TOLERATING HIS TUBE FEEDING, HE'S LETHARGIC, HASN'T URINATED ALL DAY. I TOLD HER HE WAS PROBABLY NAUSEATED FROM ULCER PAIN AND GOT A BIT DEHYDRATED, LIKE LAST TIME. ADVISED GIVING AN EXTRA DOSE OF ANTACID, AND LAYING HIM ON HIS LEFT SIDE TO NAP FOR A FEW HOURS TO SETTLE HIS STOMACH; THEN TRY CLEAR LIQUIDS FOR THE NEXT TWENTY-FOUR HOURS. MONITOR HIS HYDRATION STATUS; CALL IF IT DOESN'T IMPROVE.

And he usually did improve, so they were able to avoid another trip to the hospital.

Improve? Short-term, maybe. Long-term—never. Because Clem is Clem. Every time. Of all the children in my clinic, he takes the most work and makes the least progress. So far, I've tried to manipulate just about every aspect of his medical care—changes for the better, I thought, to simplify his routine. Tried discontinuing his medications, one by one; tried him breathing on his own without the ventilator machine; tried to teach him to hold a spoon and feed himself. I even got him fitted for eyeglasses and a hearing aid. Yet all these attempts at the fiction of making him a "more normal" little boy had failed.

So it wasn't long into managing Clem's case that I found my perspective colored by this creeping frustration. Because—I finally concluded—no matter what I do, or how hard I try, Clem is just not going to improve. His system is permanently damaged. *Permanently damaged?* You don't want to apply that label to any child, don't want to give up hope. But this is Clem. And it seemed clear that any potential for his future development was arrested long ago by the vandal meningitis infection. It's become a stalemate situation—of always reacting to a new problem, or trying to reverse a setback from an old problem—rather than making real progress.

That's my frustration.

And yet, as Clem's doctor, I'm so very far removed from it all by comparison with his mother. Which makes the puzzling phenomenon of Mrs. Knight, and her chaotic predicament, so astounding to me. I can't understand how she keeps at it, day after day, so carefully tending to him around the clock as a more-than-full-time caretaker, distraught about every minor detail in his routine. Embezzling from herself the prime era of her life to tend to this permanently flawed circumstance. With no payback—not even the ordinary rewards which make the unending struggles and sacrifices of parenting so unquestionably worthwhile: Hearing first words spoken, seeing first steps taken, feeling a soft hug around the neck, comforting hurt moist eyes looking up. Much less fulfilling any of the grander dreams which all parents have—that their child would graduate college, have success in an important career, raise a next generation of children. . . . This mother and child would cross no milestones together. Mrs. Knight would never experience the peaceful sense of respite that every parent deserves to feel at the end, after all their hard work and sacrifice—the comfort of knowing their child can make their own way to finish finding a place in the world. . . .

It's my pager beeping. "Call Dr. Carpenter in ER—*STAT*."

"This is Carpenter," he answers—"I'm calling because

Clement Knight is down here. He's your clinic patient, right? He came in about an hour ago, in bad shape. Probably another serious infection. His heart's not pumping very well, we're having a tough time keeping his blood pressure up."

"Which way do you think he's going?" I ask.

"I don't think he'll make it this time."

"Do you need some help with him?"

"Not so much with him, as with his mother. None of us can break away to talk to her about it. Can you come down and see her? We need to know his code-status—how far to go before we pull the plug. Have you two ever discussed how much she wants done for him if he came in critical?"

"No. I mean, it's never really come up between us. Is she down there now?"

"She's in the Quiet Room. I don't know how much longer we can hold on like this, before we either have to step up his support or let him go. Can you come down and ask her about it?"

"I'll sign over my patients and be right down."

My first stop—the resuscitation room where they are working on Clem. I almost can't find him on the bed, surrounded by the circle of doctors waiting in a holding pattern for further instruction. I'd never seen him without his mother at his side. He's gravely ill—ashen-colored skin, gasping, making no movement, barely any effort to breathe. His blood pressure is fluctuating borderline-low, and dropping.

Clem's in for a rough ride this time. I'd better go see Mrs. Knight right away, to negotiate this difficult situation. In most circumstances like this, it's a necessary but unjust onus to lay on a parent; to ask their wishes during a medical crisis on how far to push a resuscitation for their severely handicapped child. Most times they can't begin to answer the question, and so by default you do everything.

But this is Clem. It's not his first dire episode in critical condition. Surely Mrs. Knight had already privately considered this issue many times before. She must have prepared herself for the eventuality of it coming to this. Wouldn't she consider it to be a blessing, a benevolent "out" for all, if his incarcerated spirit was allowed to pass on? To give nature its sway to claim him, to finally free up both victim and survivors from this impossible burden? It seemed logical to me. And by their facial expressions, I deduced it also seemed logical to the other doctors who were half-resuscitating him in the other room.

But ultimately it is up to his mother.

I knock on the door to the Quiet Room. No answer. I carefully opened it—Mrs. Knight is sitting alone at the far end, facing the windowglass. She didn't turn, or look my way; seems to be distracted, more looking inward than out. I don't think she recognized my presence in the room until I stood directly in front of her.

"How is Clement?" she asks, anxiously avoiding my eyes.

"He's very sick right now. Looks like another serious infection. They've been working on him for about an hour, but he doesn't seem to be coming around. It's hard to say if he'll make it. A lot depends on how his system responds to fight it off."

Her dry, gray eyes look even further away. "He's done it before," she muttered. "I just know he'll do it this time, too."

"Mrs. Knight, there's something I need to ask you. Something personal, that we've never discussed before—because it's never really come up. It has to do with how far to take it, with Clem in critical condition like this. We call it his 'code-status.' If he gets any worse on us—can you say—do you know, I mean, *how far do you want us to*—"

She explodes out of her chair, and comes at me—turns on me, glares right into my face. Looks like she'd been ripped into by the red-hot tooth of betrayal. Transformed into an aggressive frenzy that I didn't think her capable of—a way I'd never seen her react before. And she cuts me off, like a mother cheetah protecting her litter from a pride of bigger cats—

"Of course I want everything done!"

I feel like a conspirator against her. "OK, OK," I say, trying to physically back away; but she grabs my arm, hard, and continues as if she hadn't heard me.

"Just like I did the first time he came here with meningitis. They said he wouldn't make it then, too. And how many times have we been here since? Every time I sit waiting in one of these ER rooms, I can hear them talking through the door, the other doctors in the hall saying to each other—*Oh no, not Clem again! Why don't you see him today, I had to take care of him last time.* That's *not* OK with me—for them to act like he's damaged, and don't count. Maybe he'll never be a normal little boy—but he's my miracle baby. *Now you look at me—don't you let him die! You go right back in there, and tell them I want everything done!"*

•　•　•

After teetering in critical condition in the ICU for five days, Clem's system rallied to recover. Again. On the day he went home, I heard them before I saw them. Big commotion—the staff clearing the hallway for Mrs. Knight to navigate Clem in his wide-back wheelchair, the one with the toy balloons and multicolored wheel spokes, which carried him and his life-support system out to the front of the hospital to wait for the Med Care bus.

I continued seeing Clem in my clinic throughout the rest of my residency training. Just before graduating, I passed on the responsibility for his care to a new resident. She seemed like a good listener. And for the sake of continuity, I made a photocopy of my original logbook (all except the last page), which I gave her, and reviewed with her in detail before asking if she'd definitely commit to taking him on. I made sure she understood his code status—"Full Resuscitation." And to expect that the first question Mrs. Knight would ask in clinic is whether or not the germ which caused Clem's meningitis, back when he was two months old, came from her.

Even after all these years, I still leaf through my old clinic logbook from time to time. To reread the stories of the families who helped teach me the craft of pediatrics. To remind myself of the special bond that joins them; and of the special power which all parents have, a force that makes them bigger, enables them to go far outside of themselves. I've seen it elevate the most ordinary people living everyday ordinary lives to the most fantastic feats when their child's well-being is at stake. Like the mother who stayed awake at the bedside for two straight nights to watch her baby's noisy breathing; or the parents who sold their house to pay for their boy's second bone marrow transplant; or the father who was so upset when his seven-year-old son Zack was afraid to go to school because the others might tease him after he lost all his hair from the chemotherapy, so the father shaved his own head bald and told the boy he did it so he could be just like his hero, Zack. . . .

Then I finish by reading the quote I'd written on the last page of my logbook; the one I've privately referred to many times throughout my career. Which says: "To work and to love"—the reply Sigmund Freud made at the end of his life and long career, when asked: "What is the key to personal fulfillment?"

"To work and to love." I didn't copy that page from the logbook for the resident who took over Clem's care, because I thought she should come to her own conclusions. I don't recall what prompted me to write it there in the first place; but I do remember I was thinking about *heroism* at the time. About having the courage to make an ultimate sacrifice in this life; to stand up for something good, believe in it so completely that you will do whatever it takes to make it count. Which is what being a parent raising a child is all about. *Any* child. It's hoisting them up on your shoulders to see the parade pass by; sometimes it's hanging toy balloons on an iron lung. One of the few, almost impossible privileges we get to go beyond our mortal, flawed, and otherwise insignificant lives, to touch a hand on something infinite.

The pediatrican's job is to help facilitate this privilege. It usually doesn't take much—because there is no force in all creation more powerful or compelling or inspiring than a mother urging the needs of her child; except the mother who has devoted her life to urging the special needs of her handicapped child.

Each parent has a right to insist on telling the story their own way: To handle it, shape it, even make it noble—to register its legitimacy in the log of humanity. Whenever I see these mysterious urgings being played out, I wonder at it more because I understand it less, and find I can never take it for granted.

Joker Card

A tranquil Sunday morning so far in the ER. *Almost* tranquil. There's more housekeeping than medicine being practiced—nurses restock rooms with equipment and linens, janitors vacuum and mop, secretaries file paperwork. No patients presenting—yet. A bonus morning for me, I get a chance to catch up: Sort through mail, scan medical journals, return phone calls. Yet it's never really tranquil, because you are always waiting, even during a lull like this—always on alert for the next emergency to burst through the door which requires the immediate attention of an ER doctor.

ER doctor. After finishing my residency training in pediatrics, I chose to work in the emergency room at Children's Hospital. I like the fast-paced action, juggling a variety of difficult medical problems, trying to make order out of chaos. It takes all your concentration, working ER—demands you be ready to react at every moment of your shift. Even during a Sunday morning lull like this. Because anything can present at any time. The next case coming through the door could be a toothache or an amputation. Or both. And you often get only one "best" chance at managing it.

Time for coffee. My morning comfort. Brewing in the nurses' dinner-break room. For some odd reason, the hospital decided to mount the x-ray viewbox back here—the rectangular metal box with an opaque glass front and a light inside, used to illuminate x-ray films for our inspection. ER doctors are not radiologists—except after-hours and on weekends, when the radiologist is off—and then we have to read our patients' x-rays. Seems this dusty old viewbox has always been back here. I can't figure out why; it only makes it more difficult to concentrate on reading a film when the room is full of people who are eating and talking and laughing.

As I fill my cup with hot black coffee, I notice there is some morning housekeeping for me, too—an x-ray, hanging on the unlit viewbox; which probably wasn't returned to the radiology department after the ER doctor inspected it last night. I can't see the detail of the unlit film. . . .

I remove the x-ray to place it in the outbox. The snap sound made by pulling on the plastic sheet with my fingers, the tactile sensation of holding the smooth-edged black and white negative film in my hand, my proximity to the unlit viewbox, the scent of brewing coffee . . . prompts an impulse, an automatic reflex that's urged me thousands of times before: *Data. Interpret. Challenge.* It's part of the continual process of molting your former self as you evolve your skills.

Look at it. I automatically flick the film back up onto the viewbox glass, and click on the light beneath. My eyes are driven to scan it methodically, my brain to reconstruct the two-dimensional picture into the three-dimensionality of real anatomy. What I see links up, with best fit, to a like image stored in my mental file of x-ray patterns: It's a side view of the neck—of an older child, judging from the size of the bones, probably a teenager. The name printed on the film is "Lu Wong"; it was performed at 11:22 P.M. last night.

The neck has seven vertebral bones, the upper "back bones," stacked in a column one on top of another. Like solid white rings of smoke, spanning from the bottom of the skull down to the top of the shoulders. They are the support casing around the tender spinal cord—tender, with the consistency of gelatin—yet so important, the electric highway carrying the life signals for movement from the brain to the muscles of the body. Each bony ring is connected to the one above and below by tough ligaments and joints and muscle, forming a strong yet flexibly bonded system. A marvel of evolutionary architecture, like the bird feather—protective, lightweight, supple, durable. The straight and true alignment of these bones protects the cord from traumatic injury and shock. Any disruption of this alignment can cause pressure, bruising, bleeding, even severance of the cord.

A severed cord in the neck is the most devastating of injuries—an utter catastrophe—because it causes immediate, permanent paralysis of the body's musculature. The patient can't move anything from the neck down—for life. The prevention of which is one of the most dramatically important duties of an ER doctor.

My scanning snags on something abnormal at the top—*right here*—the second vertebral bone is slightly tilted forward, out of alignment with the bones above and below it, because of—it's subtle—because of the tiny hairline crack right through here. *Is this a fracture? No—can't be.* But it sure looks like a "Hangman's" fracture. A rare injury in children, one I've only seen a few times—called "Hangman's" because it's the type of neck fracture which occurs after a long drop through a gallows floor with the noose tucked under the chin, as perfected by the British penal system. Or the type of injury anyone can sustain when the top of their head slams into a solid surface. *Is it?* The fine tremor in my hand holding my coffee cup is telling me that *yes—it's a "Hangman's."*

Start over. I have to look away, then back again, to refocus my eyes, to corroborate every detail. *Look here*—a hairline crack through the back of the bone; *and here*—another, just beneath. And look at how the vertebrae are slightly out of alignment—now I'm sure it's a "Hangman's."

Surely this fracture was recognized last night, and this patient was admitted to ICU by a neurosurgeon. Yet ICU always keeps the x-rays of their patients up in their unit. Why is it still here?

I need more information—need to check Lu Wong's medical record from last night. I quickly sort through the pile of 100 or so ER charts of patients seen during the past twenty-four hours. "Wong"—it sounds like a Southeast-Asian Hmong name. *Vang, Xiong, Chang. . . .* There it is—second from the last chart in the pile. Sure enough—it states she was—*sent home!* No doubt it is her—Lu Wong—the diagnosis written is "Passenger—motor vehicle accident—sprained neck." No mention of a fracture. The state patrol snapped a polaroid of the car wreck—it shows a spidery crack in the windshield on the passenger side where her head struck. The point of impact that might very well have changed her life forever.

Who saw her? The physician's signature at the bottom of the chart shows it was Marcus. *Marcus?* He's usually so thorough—someone I routinely ask to help *me* read difficult x-rays. How did he miss it? And yet on a busy ER shift you only get about ten seconds to inspect an x-ray. Ten seconds—then have to move on to other waiting business. Maybe during that ten seconds he let up, relaxed the focus of his concentration, or was distracted by some other activity going on around him; and blanked-out seeing the fracture. Or maybe he misjudged the full extent of this patient's symptoms. The Hmong can be very stoic; it's partly due to a mistrust of Western medicine, partly caused by the confusion of translating languages. I've seen Hmong stoicism many times; the children never cry, they stare straight ahead and don't react even with starting an IV or performing a spinal tap. Almost as if it is unforgivably shameful to act up in public. After a while you come to expect it, adjust for it.

But a broken neck? The books teach there should be some obvious sign—severe pain, severe limitation in the neck's range of motion, weakness in the hands and feet—something to indicate more than just a sprain. *What else did Mark write?* Says here: *"The patient has slight neck pain, which improved during her ER stay; she moves her arms and legs, walks normally. No complaint of headache or weakness.*" All usually reliable signs to predict a low risk for fracture.

One last look . . . no; the x-ray hasn't changed, won't transform to normal—the fracture is still there. If this were my patient, I would be running back to her exam room to hold her head steady, until the neurosurgeon came to take her to surgery to wire the fractured bones. But she's not my patient. Actually, she just became my patient—and I know what I have to do: Contact this family, tell them what has happened to their daughter; make them keep her motionless until the paramedics come and transport her back to the ER. Hopefully the fractured area is still providing enough support and stability to prevent damage to the tender, irreparable spinal cord tissue. Her straining too hard, bending down to tie her shoes, even a harmless sneeze, could instantly transform her from a fully-mobile, fully-functioning young person with a limitless future of motion—to the flaccid confinement of a wheelchair-bound quadriplegic.

It's 7:30 A.M. The Wong home phone number is listed on the chart. I dial it quickly. Someone should be there on this early Sunday morning. I have to convey urgency without panic, persuade them to keep her as still and quiet as possible until the paramedics arrive. Hopefully she hasn't sneezed—

The phone rings and rings. And rings. No answer. I wish this was a cordless phone, I really need to get up and pace. After several minutes of more ringing, I hang up and then redial, hoping I misdialed the first time. It continues ringing—still no answer. I have visions of a catastrophe on the other end: That a healthy, active teenage girl with a whole life of good health ahead of her made a move, or strained herself in an otherwise harmless way, and is now lying senseless on the floor. All of which was preventable.

Come on, come on. Somebody pick up the phone. Still no answer.

What now? I redial the number every ten minutes for the next hour. Each time it just rings. I'd get in my car and drive to their house, if I could . . . but it's my shift today, and the charts of new patients waiting to be seen are starting to pile up on the counter. What if any of *them* is really sick and needs my full attention?

At 8:30 A.M., I call the police.

"Dispatch officer. How can I help you?"

"This is Children's Hospital Emergency Room calling. We need your help. Got a serious situation—a child seen here last night who was sent home with a broken neck. I've been calling the family all morning to get them back here, but no one answers the phone. I'm hoping they're still asleep. Can you send a squad car out right away to rouse these people? Tell the officers that if they get in to keep everyone calm, and call 911 for the paramedics."

"OK. I'm sending a unit."

My next responsibility is to call Marcus, since the outcome of this could impact on his career. He could lose his medical license if this patient has a bad outcome after leaving his care in the ER last night. Even if legally able to practice, the psychological damage done to an ER doctor's confidence after a case like this can be irreparable. More than one is disabled.

I put the call in to him. It's a difficult call to make. Because we've been friends for a long time—went through medical school and residency training together. Worked ER side by side for years now. It's a difficult call to make, because I have to tell him something that I know will hurt him. And because making a call like this is a reminder—that someday I might be on the receiving end of a call like this. Might be? *Will* be. It's inevitable—every ER doctor has at least one nightmare story to tell. About the one you missed. You can't get through an ER career without it happening at least once. It's a price you pay, working in this field—and you carry it with you for the rest of your life. Knowing that you were put in charge, and missed something—something important—either because of inexperience, or because you were tired at the end of a busy shift and your concentration slipped, or just because you were dealt the joker card that day. You worry about it happening every time you pick up a new chart.

Now it's Marcus' turn. Which makes it a difficult call to make. When you get the call it feels like the floor's dropped out and you're in a howling free-fall. With everybody watching your descent. I know what has to be said, but not quite how to say it. I need to use my "breaking bad news" doctor tact, even on a fellow practitioner—sound calm, as if every detail is being attended to; supportive, without being judgmental. He must be involved in the decision making if he wants to be, because it's his career in jeopardy—

"Hello."

"Mark? Hi—hope I'm not calling too early. Did I wake you?"

"No. I'm up. Working at the computer. What's going on? Sounds like you're at work."

"I've got the day shift today."

"I was on last night," he said. "Till after midnight. Long shift. Really busy."

It's best to push right into it—"Mark, I'm calling to get some information. Do you remember seeing a teenage patient last night named Lu Wong? The chart says 'female involved in a motor vehicle accident.' Looks like she was here about 11 P.M.?"

Those words—*do you remember seeing a patient*—it's the last thing you want to hear on the day after a busy shift. It almost always means you missed something important. You know what comes next, after *do you remember seeing a patient.* . . . Which is why I don't feel like much of a friend now, because I can spot him moving like a target into the crosshairs.

"Car accident—right? Yeah. Sprained neck, I think. I did an x-ray, and sent her home—*right?*" After a short pause, his voice sounded different. *"Why? Is anything wrong?"*

"I stumbled onto her x-ray this morning, it was on the viewbox in the back. And I think I see something abnormal."

"Abnormal? What abnormal?" his voice groped, like someone in a dark room trying to put a hand on a wall. Any wall.

"It's a serious injury to the neck. Looks like a fracture."

"No. *No.*" It doesn't sound like Mark anymore. I can see him recoiling on the other end of the telephone line. "No—can't be. Are you sure it's my patient? Now I remember—she had hardly any neck pain. It got better before she went home. I know, because I examined her twice. Three times. She moved her arms and legs, walked without any problem. Are you sure she's my patient?"

"Yes. It's your signature at the bottom of the chart."

"And you saw the film?"

"I have it here in front of me." I have to be firm with him at this point, so he understands and follows and we can move on. "It's a fracture. Looks like a 'Hangman's.' Been calling the family all morning to get her back here, but so far no answer. Got the police working on it. Hopefully they'll make contact with them."

"My signature? Are you sure? My x-ray? I always scan them more than once, just to make sure. But I was exhausted at the end of the shift last night—did I really pass right over it?"

Exhausted . . . passed right over it. . . . That kind of fatigue is routine at the end of a busy ER shift. When you almost can't focus your eyes anymore, and everyone else needs something— nurses firing requests: *The diabetic in Room Y needs insulin orders written before he gets his snack; the asthmatic in Room B is wheezing again, can you take a listen and say whether she needs another aerosol treatment?; we're all set up for you to stitch the cut in Room D; by the way, that dehydrated toddler in Room F pulled out his IV, and none of us can get another one in—when can you give it a try?; the mother in Room G has a few questions about her son's operation in the morning, whenever you have time. . . .* Then your pager beeps for an outside phone call when you're halfway through stitching the cut in Room D—it's the endocrinologist, asking for report on the diabetic in Room Y:

Did he get his snack yet? How much insulin did you give? While other doctors hold on blinking phone lines, crabby because you woke them to discuss their patient. And another wave of new patients is waiting to be seen, with frustrated parents standing in the doorway of their rooms watching your every move, wondering—*"when is it our turn?"*—

All while you try to concentrate for ten seconds on reading an x-ray. *Passed right over it* is bound to occur. Like driving half-asleep and forgetting a stretch of dark highway. All ER doctors miss things from time to time—but it's usually a minor issue, like a hairline fracture of a finger or toe; something that can be safely followed up on the next day. But this scenario is an ER doctor's worst nightmare: A patient is entrusted to your care with a serious, life-threatening injury who arrives in stable condition; you get your chance at it, but miss—and they are sent home. Then the nightmare—the patient decompensates; in this case the "decompensation" being complete and permanent paralysis below the neck. Left to steer a wheelchair by blowing through a straw.

"Mark, if you want to come in and manage this I'll be glad to help out."

I am obliged to make the offer, since it's his career on the line. But I hope he doesn't take me up on it—because he has a personal stake in this case now. Working ER, you learn to hand off to your doctor-partner when you are in over your head. Like he is now. I want to say something to nudge him in that direction; he probably feels embarrassed, thinks he made a mess that someone else has to clean up—

"It's been quiet here so far this morning; and I feel like I'm on top of the situation," I said, glancing at the thickening stack of new charts piling up on the counter.

"OK then. The family probably wouldn't want me involved in the case now, anyway. You let me know what's going on."

The ER secretary motions to me. "It's the police on the line for you."

"Got to go, it's the police calling. Maybe they made contact with the family. I'll call back."

I punch the blinking button. It's the dispatch officer.

"Yes doctor, we sent a squad car to the Wong house but no one is there. The officers tried the doors and windows—no answer. They told the neighbors to watch for them. A squad will cruise back in thirty minutes to try again."

I have visions of a teenage girl with a severed spinal cord, who is collapsed and lying motionless on the floor, breathlessly unable to summon help. Should I ask the officers to break down the door and search the premises?

The ER secretary motions to me again. "A call on line one."

It's Marcus. "What did the police say?"

"Nobody home. Got the neighbors watching for them."

"I just can't believe this is happening," he said. "I've dreaded this my whole career. I try so hard to be careful, to make sure . . . then this happens. I'll be home all day. Call me with any news."

I'm back to calling the Wongs', redialing their number every ten minutes or so. While it's ringing, I quickly scan through the pile of new charts on the counter; none of the patients' complaints seem to be too serious—sore throat, twisted ankle, ear pain . . . certainly nothing as serious as this. They will have to wait. We are all waiting.

10:30 A.M. The ringing of the phone is constant in my ear. Then it stops. *Am I disconnected?* After an infinite moment of silence, unbelievably, there is a sleepy female voice on the other end.

"Hello?"

"Yes—hello? Yes—this is the doctor from Children's Hospital—"

Slow down, don't talk so fast, get control. "I'm trying to reach the parents of Lu Wong, a patient seen here in the emergency room last night. Are you her mother?"

"No."

"Who are you?"

"I'm Lu."

There's hot panic expanding in my chest—because to answer the phone she must be up and moving around. Up, and moving—which is the last thing I want.

"You are Lu Wong?"

"Yes."

"Were you in a car accident last night?"

"Yes."

"Were you seen here in the ER last night?"

"Yes."

"OK. I'm calling to—to see how you are doing today. How are you doing? How is your neck?"

"It hurt all night. It hurts now. Why? What's wrong?"

"We have a question about your x-ray from last night. So we need to examine you again this morning. Is anyone else there with you?"

"My brother."

"How old is he?"

"Eighteen."

"Where are your parents?"

"I think they went to the vegetable market."

"Let me talk to your brother. I want you to hand him the phone, then go lie down on your back, flat on the floor—look straight up at the ceiling, and don't move or get up. Do you understand?"

"OK. Hang on."

"Hello?"

"Yes. This is the doctor from Children's Hospital. Are you Lu's brother?"

"Yes."

"What's your name?"

"Vu."

"OK, Vu. Listen carefully. We've got a serious problem, and I'm counting on you to help manage it."

"What's wrong?"

"Your sister has a serious injury to her neck. We need to get her back to the ER right away. Safely. So you have to do exactly as I say."

"OK. What do I have to do?"

"Is she lying flat on the floor?"

"Yes."

"Looking straight up?"

"Yes."

"OK. I'm going to call the paramedics. They'll come to get her. When I hang up, go open the door. Then kneel next to your sister and hold her head straight with the rest of her body. Head looking up. Do not let her move or turn or get up or go to the bathroom or eat anything. Just keep her as still as possible until the paramedics get there. Don't let her sneeze."

"What?"

"Just hold her head straight until the paramedics get there. Stay calm, I don't want her to get upset—OK?"

"OK."

After the 911 call, I sit for a moment to catch my breath. *Did I forget anything?* Time to call Mark.

"Mark—good news so far—I made contact. The girl actually answered the phone. She sounded good. The paramedics are going to get her now. How are you doing?"

"Terrible. I can't sit still—been pacing and sweating all morning. My wife knows something is wrong, but I just can't talk to her about it. So the girl is on her way back?"

"Right. I'll call you again after I examine her."

Now there are *two* stacks of new charts piled on the counter. The ER's backed up a full three hours. No time to worry about that. I hurried off to the ambulance bay area just outside the ER to wait. To meet them as they pull up and supervise her transport. There's certainly nothing hectic about the peaceful Sunday morning blue out here, or the quiet row of rooks perched in judgment on a powerline overhead. Off in the distance, I hear the slowly building crescendo of a siren navigating the gridwork of city streets. Coming closer. If that's her being conveyed, at least her neck has been immobilized in a brace by the paramedics—and whatever damage which might have occurred as a result of her leaving here last night is stabilized. . . .

The ambulance slowly taxies under the canopy of the ER entrance. The reverse-direction warning bell tolls as it docks in front of the door. I want to jump up on the rig and take over. *Don't—hold off, for just a bit longer.* The transport isn't quite completed; best to let due process take its course.

Two brawny paramedics carefully unload the girl from the rig on a stretcher at a slow, methodical pace. *Be careful. Roll the cart smoothly.* I cringe each time they hit a bump. She's lying flat, strapped to a wooden backboard securing her body— head and neck and shoulders—wearing a rigid plastic brace wrapped tightly around the neck and tucked under the chin. A sandbag on each side of her head to stabilize it in place. Her brother follows the stretcher. At first it's a relief to see that she looks almost comfortable; but then again, she is Hmong.

Now it's up to physics and luck and fate. As they wheel her into her the ER, I see she can move her arms and legs, her fingers; she's taking full breaths. No obvious sign of paralysis. I have to corroborate this by thoroughly examining every minute aspect of her neurologic function.

The paramedics transfer her on the backboard to the hospital bed. Now she is mine to manage. There's no expression of pain or discomfort on her face. I can't tell by looking at her that there's anything wrong, much less that she has a broken neck. She makes no reaction when I lightly press over the fractured area. Strength, sensation, motor function, reflexes—all normal. All aspects of her neurologic exam are miraculously normal.

. . .

Just after I complete my exam, the family arrives and silently engulfs the room. The good thing about Hmong families is everyone comes during a medical crisis. The bad thing about Hmong families is everyone comes during a medical crisis. Grandparents, cousins, neighbors, the shaman medicine man— all generations, from infants to elders. With bags and bags of vegetables from the morning market. Seems the entire Hmong community is quickly mobilized through some secret underground network, and they all come, every time. All standing here now in silent witness, as if the mass of their hushed presence had the power to heal.

The immediate family is identified by their closest proximity to the patient's bed. The father stands barely five feet tall; is bony-thin, wiry, bow-legged, with stringy jet-black hair. His sallow complexion and chiseled facial bones could be mistaken for Native American on a larger body frame. The clothing tattered but clean. He appears to be a first-generation Hmong immigrant, who barely speaks broken English; yet by the intensity of his eyes I can tell he is bright and perceptive. I've learned it is the Hmong father who makes the important decisions in the Hmong family.

I introduce myself and prepare to explain step-by-step what has happened. In situations like this you come to understand just how different working ER is from private practice—because, often on a moment's notice, you must deal with families in crisis who don't know you. And have to develop an instant rapport which allows them to trust you to assume the care of their sick or injured child. I feel disadvantaged in this particular situation, because instead of just representing myself, I am more the embodiment of all Western medicine to them—and of all ER doctors.

What if the father asks about the missed fracture last night? What should I say? That sometimes these things happen—but it's rare? Will that satisfy? One in a million odds is no comfort to a parent when their child is the one afflicted.

"We brought your daughter back this morning because it looks like there's a broken bone in her neck on the x-ray from last night."

I catch myself inanely raising my voice to him, as if increasing the volume of English somehow improves its translation to a foreigner.

"We were careful to bring her back right away, so a spine doctor can treat her. The good news is her exam is normal, I don't see any sign of injury to the spinal cord. I think she is going to do very well."

I search the father's face for his reaction. Even though he seems to follow the logic of my argument, there is no eye contact made, no dialogue between us, no sense of relief expressed in his demeanor. He stares right past me—his eyes are focused on something else, far off—he seems to be skeptical, as if waiting for something more.

Perhaps he will better comprehend all of this if I show him the x-ray from last night, and point out the fracture—

"Come in the back room with me, sir, and let me show you the x-ray."

I flick the film onto the lit viewbox. To elucidate the anatomic details, the faint hairline fracture, the slight degree of bony malalignment. Seeing the data can help give a parent an appreciation for just how difficult it is to identify these subtle abnormalities. And hearing the technical medical jargon can instill confidence in the doctor's capability.

But before I can go any further, the father's face flushes with anger—anger and frustration. His moistened yellowed eyes glisten intently on the glowing metal box. He closes them. He opens them. Then speaks, for the first time:

"I tol docta eet bruk. Heem no leesen. Eet bruk—rat de."

And he reaches up his short, thin, gnarled index finger, like a divining rod, and points to the exact location of the "Hangman's" fracture.

"Heem no leesen. I tol heem eet bruk. Heem no leesen."

I am dumbstruck. Should I laugh now, or just go home? Did I actually hear him say what I thought I heard him say? If I did, then *how could he know that?* I almost slipped, and asked him . . . but caught myself in time. You can't ask—because asking can open a dangerous door, an invitation for him to expand on his anger; which could then undermine my control in managing this case. I need to compose myself—because at this point I'm in the unusual and awkward position of having absolutely nothing further to say or do.

Fortunately my pager beeps me out of the room for a phone call. After leaving, I scan the personal information section of Lu Wong's chart; under "Father's Occupation" is written "chicken farmer."

It's Marcus. "Did she get there? What happened? Did you see her? How is she?"

"Everything is OK, her exam is normal, she looks good."

"Say it again."

"Everything is normal. The neurosurgeon is here. He's taking her to surgery to wire the bones together."

"*Normal.* I can't believe it. There's nothing normal about the past twelve hours of my life. Twelve hours? It feels more like a twenty-year stretch. Been sitting here worrying, wondering about the rest of my life. Thinking that if she came back injured I would have quit ER. Even quit medicine. How could I ever be responsible for another important case after dropping the ball like that? Is the family there?"

"They're all here."

"Are they mad about what happened last night?"

"I think they're relieved she's OK."

"You know," he said, "I've been thinking and thinking all morning: *What went wrong? What did I miss?* And then I remembered something—weird—that happened with this case last night. Really weird. When I told the family the x-ray was normal, the shaman began rubbing coins on the girl's arms and legs. Then the father put his hand on her neck, and closed his eyes. After about a minute, he looked up at me and said *no, her neck is broken.* I couldn't believe it, I thought it was some kind of joke. Never had anything like it happen before. It caught me off guard, and I guess I just kept going. I probably should have stopped, and listened more carefully."

Making order out of chaos. You have the front-line responsibility for diagnosing and managing thousands of ill and injured patients who come in off the street during your ER career.

Accurately, efficiently, compassionately. No matter how tired, or what your mood, or what else is going on around you. It takes many years to accept the lonely fact that you can never be perfect at it. Even though you play at high stakes, and others expect infallibility, and even though you get better at it each time, eventually you come to understand there are many factors outside your control which determine the outcome of any case. Sometimes—even though you do your best to prepare, and use all your knowledge and experience in proceeding—sometimes your number is called, and that day you get dealt the joker card.

When it happens, all you can hope is that something else comes along—some odd piece of information, a subtle clue, a quirky hunch—from somewhere, to snag your attention and help clarify what's unfolding before it's too late.

There is a certain *something*—call it insight, intuition, clairvoyance—call it what you will, it's not listed in the index of any medical textbook. Yet I've encountered it enough times to know it's a real thing. Powerful. Especially the kind of synchronicity binding a parent to their child. Parents know certain things about their children in a way the doctor can never know. It's inscrutable. The closest thing in this life to merging two separate and distinct realities into one—perhaps because they aren't so very separate and distinct after all.

Each time I encounter it working ER revalidates the lesson: Take time to stop, and listen carefully; maintain vigilance for that crucial piece of information which can come from anywhere at any time. Especially when a parent has a hunch about their child. It can help to clarify, help to guide—if you let it. Even when it comes from the most unlikely source—like at the end of the gnarled twisted pointing-finger of an immigrant father's intuition.

Wings of Wax

AUGUST 11, 1992
THE EMERGENCY ROOM
CHILDREN'S HOSPITAL

The dispatch radio crackles. An ambulance call is coming in over the speaker.

"This is Medic Transport calling Children's Hospital ER. Come in, Children's."

There's a split second of siren noise in the background for as long as the paramedic voice is on. Sirens always grab your attention. But sirens are generic. So everyone within earshot stops their business for a moment, to hear how serious a thing is coming. Could be anything from constipation to a full cardiac arrest. I'm guessing constipation, or the like, because the voice on the other end sounds detached and unhurried.

A nurse picks up the radio receiver. "Go ahead Medic, this is Children's."

"We are en route with a fourteen-year-old female. Suicide attempt. Ingested ten acetaminophen tablets. She vomited once. Her vital signs are stable. We should be there in a few minutes."

"Copy, Medic. We'll be waiting. Out." The nurse hangs up, and writes the information in the log. Then turns to us, and discreetly repeats the report: "Teenager, suicide attempt, took ten acetaminophen tablets, transport is a few minutes out . . ." just loud enough to be heard by the other ER staff without the information spilling over into the exam rooms.

Another teenager-ingestion case. Just managed one, about a week ago. Same thing: A girl who took a handful of pills—iron pills, I think. Luckily, everything turned out OK. I remember after we finished our medical management I found myself standing there, looking at her lying on the bed withdrawn and remorseful, and I was curious as to why a young person with their whole life ahead of them would do something like that— try to harm themselves. So I asked her—*why?* And she said she wasn't really trying to kill herself, she just got mad when her mother wouldn't let her buy the clothes she needed to start school. *Over school clothes?* My reflex reaction was to think— *how ridiculous.* It was the only reaction I could muster after seeing so many other sick kids, like kids with terminal cancer, who would give anything for just another year of school, never mind the wardrobe. But later, after considering it further, I was reminded that clothing to a teenager goes far beyond just a superficial something to wear; it's the emblem of how they relate to their peers. *Which, to her at the time, was everything.* Sometimes it's not easy, but you have to find a way to under- stand and respect their perspective if you are to make progress and move ahead with a teen.

. . .

Today it's an acetaminophen ingestion. Which can be very serious, even fatal, because an overdose can destroy the liver. No need for panic—not yet—only ten acetaminophen tablets ingested by a teenager *shouldn't* cause serious toxicity. *Shouldn't.* But—you always have to qualify—that's if she actually took *only ten* tablets. I've managed teens who said they took ten pills when they actually took one hundred and ten. So you never know for sure until you confirm it with a blood test. And then there is the possibility of a "surprise" co-ingestion—that she took something else with the acetaminophen, and didn't tell—something much more dangerous, like an antidepressant medication which can cause seizures, coma, even cardiac arrest and sudden death. . . .

There are always many unanswered questions early in the course of a case like this. Which is why we initiate the "ingestion protocol" when they arrive; because in most cases, the more time that elapses before treatment, the greater the risk for serious toxicity. We have to get set up, there is much to do.

"Can you take this girl when she comes in?" I ask the nurse who answered the radio call.

"Joan and I can get her going."

"OK. Start the decontamination. Then I'll be in to examine her."

The nurses dress in their waterproof gowns, plastic goggles, face masks, bouffant surgical hats, rubber gloves. It always looks like they are about to enter a biohazard waste site. Which is usually what the room becomes after the decontamination procedure is finished.

• • •

The sliding glass doors open down the hall, and the paramedics wheel the gurney toward us at a slow pace.

"Where do you want her?" they ask.

"Let's go into Room B. We're all set up."

The girl is a young teenager. More young than teen. Still in that awkward braces-on-her-teeth phase. Rings on each finger, glitter nail polish. She looks withdrawn and frightened, like all the others once they are wheeled into the ER. The expression on their faces is always the same—once they see the nurses dressed like alien space travelers, and the room set up with tubes and bags of saline and the jumbo syringes, and the IV kit, and the monitors lit and beeping. For the first time it registers that there is a lot more going to happen here than they first expected.

The paramedics transfer her to the hospital bed in Room B, and exit to finish their paperwork.

"What's the story?" I ask them in the hallway.

"Don't know. She wouldn't talk to us."

"Where's mom?"

"In registration. She rode with us in the rig. She knows we're in here, and that you're going to get started."

The nurses close the door to Room B, so the girl can change into a hospital gown and they can begin the decontamination. In the meantime I'll write orders, then go in to examine her. I'm more likely to get honest answers to my questions if I'm not perceived as party to the upcoming painful procedure. Questions—to determine whether this is a true suicide attempt. Most times it isn't; most teenagers who take a handful of pills are seeking attention and don't actually intend to harm themselves. It's not a true "suicide attempt"; it's termed a "suicide *gesture*," or an "adolescent *adjustment-reaction*." The distinction is important, because "gesture" and "adjustment-reaction" imply they aren't likely to repeat the act. I'll ask the questions, but it will be up to a psychiatrist to make the final determination. After we manage the medical part, they come in to evaluate the psychological part.

Psychological part. Some of my most difficult ER cases are teens. That compelling mix of body and desire and curiosity and appetite, all of which is too commonly fast-forwarded past the ability to gauge and measure and judge. Teens are physically capable of doing adult-type things which can alter the course of many lives—like fostering children, or disabling themselves under the dark cloak of addiction, or exerting enough force to maim or kill. . . . You have to remind yourself when managing a difficult teen case that desire is not tempered by reason; and that, often at this age, everything moves in one heady direction and at one hectic speed.

You never forget the difficult teens in this business. Risk-takers—drug overdose, venereal disease, unplanned pregnancy. The contradiction of a child doing harm to themselves and closing doors to their future is so foreign to the rest of your pediatric experience. The main reason I chose a career in pediatrics (and not adult medicine) is because the medical problems of children are rarely, if ever, due to self-abuse or negligence. So your doctoring effort is focused on the more meaningful end of correcting an honest mistake, or reversing a natural calamity.

Yet somewhere during the teen years the pediatric line is crossed. Like the sixteen-year-old asthmatic who didn't refill his prescriptions for six months, and was carried into the ER almost asphyxiated from wheezing; then, after we worked on him for five days in the ICU (he was on a breathing machine for three of them) and finally got his lungs cleared and sent him home, I saw him loitering with his friends at the mall—*smoking cigarettes.* Or the teenage boy who lost a precious index finger and suffered a severe burn to his face and chest when a bottle-rocket went off in his hand. Or the covered body of a teenage "John Doe" drunk driver, who you were asked to formally pronounce dead and call the coroner for. . . .

It's always a difficult sell on my part—offering "counsel" to a teenager to see it as otherwise. To expect they will consider the notion of "cause and effect," resist acting on their urges, or temporize based on an understanding of "limitation." *Limitation?* Not likely, when at that age there has been no sense of the sad regret which comes after you've done something to permanently close a door in this life.

So today it's an acetaminophen ingestion. The first priority is gastrointestinal decontamination. Gut clean out. A flush job, in two phases. Phase one is gastric lavage—pumping the stomach—using a three-foot-long rigid plastic tube (it looks like a garden hose) which is passed through the mouth and down the esophagus; then the tube is flushed, in and out, with saline solution until clear of all pill fragments. Phase two—the patient drinks the binding agent, which flushes through the intestines to capture and eliminate any drug left over in the bowel.

It's been a quiet ten minutes in Room B, I haven't heard any noise from within. Which usually indicates the lavage went smoothly. After logging my orders in the computer, I enter; the girl is dressed in a hospital gown, sitting stiffly upright on the bed, looking down at the large plastic basin on her lap used to catch the expelled vomitus. Yet the basin is dry and empty. One nurse is poised holding an unused lavage tube, the other waiting with a saline flush. *Why haven't they begun?*

"How's it going?" I ask.

"We're having a little trouble negotiating the tube going down."

"Need some help?"

"Sure."

I put on rubber gloves, and introduce myself to the girl. She stares down into the empty basin.

"Do you understand everything we have to do, and why?" I ask her.

She looks distant, but quietly panicked. She makes no eye contact, gives no response.

Seems I always get the urge to preach at a time like this, out of frustration, when a teenager doesn't seem to make any attempt to cooperate. I want to say something obvious, like "You realize this is the consequence of your actions," or "You might think about this next time," or. . . . But I resist the urge. Partly because it never has any meaningful effect. And because I don't want to add the degradation of shame to what comes next— the stinging pain she's about to experience when I pass that long rigid tube down her throat. I don't want to do it; inflicting pain on a child goes against my doctor's instinct. But the medical reality here dictates it must be done.

Better pause for a moment before we get started, to make sure she understands what is coming next, and why.

"As your doctor, I need to tell you a few things about all this. What you did could be very serious. Some people think acetaminophen isn't dangerous because you can buy it over the counter. But you need to know that an overdose can destroy the liver. And you can't live without a liver. I'm not saying this just to scare you; we'll be able to tell how serious it is from the blood test. But it's important information for you to think about next time, before you decide to act like this."

She makes no reaction to my empty lecture. Time to get on with the lavage.

"So we have to empty out your stomach with the tube. Do you understand?"

She barely nods, without looking up.

"It takes about a minute to get the tube down. It's uncomfortable. You'll gag; probably throw up. But it'll go quickly if you take slow deep breaths. You'll still be able to breathe even though it feels like you are choking. Try not to fight it. If you fight, it's more difficult. Sorry we have to do this."

We always work from both sides of the bed with the patient facing forward because of what's to come. I use my left hand to firmly hold the girl's head back against the upright-positioned top of the bed. She cooperates by opening her mouth. I use my right hand to pass the tube.

Once it's on her tongue there's nothing she can do to stop

it. It's always a painful few minutes for everyone—the assault—because when the tip grates against the back of her throat, she starts to gag, then retch, the kind of deep awful whole-body gut retching made to expel a menacingly noxious thing. I have to push the tube hard at first, so the tip can make the sharp turn down the back of her throat. Then come the dark muffled coughs and choking sounds, like the panicked scream of someone submerged and drowning; muffled, because the large-diameter tube is pushing against her vocal cords.

The girl bites down hard on the tube, her only defense against the stabbing pain running through the middle of her body. She can't bite while gagging, so I advance it further with each choke-spasm. When it's about halfway down, she starts to vomit—up and out—volumes of partially digested food, bile, and brown curdled liquid mixed with white pill fragments splatter into the basin. More and more comes up, up and out. Her choking vibrates through the liquidity. The soured rotten stench of it fills the room, taints the air—which is nauseating, makes me feel sick inside like vomiting too. I want to turn away, but have to keep pushing. She vomits up and out through the tube, around the tube, out through her nose—some hits in the basin, some on her lap, some on the bed and the floor. A lot ends up on my arm and hand pushing the tube; I almost lose my grip because it's slippery-wet to hold with a soiled rubber glove. Just a bit more to go—

She panics and struggles with having her head restrained through the choking and pain, so I have to hold just a bit more firmly. Otherwise, the reflex to protect herself will cause her to grab the tube and yank it out. And then we would have to start all over. Her nostrils are flared wide; her fingers gripping my arm are white-hot with tension. I hold her head more firmly— yet try to reassure her that she won't suffocate, to take slow deep breaths. *Breathe through your nose,* I say. Her eyes well up full from the stinging pain. One more push—there it is—the yellow stomach juice refluxing back through the tube signifies it is in place.

"That's all—it's in. No more pushing," I tell her. "Take a deep breath. Are you OK?"

She barely nods.

"We'll hold the tube right here. No more pushing. Just take slow deep breaths. OK—let's do the lavage."

Her eyes dart back and forth to see what is coming next. I loosen my grip on her head a bit, and anchor the tube in place by holding it down against the inner surface of her lower front teeth. The nurse begins the lavage, flushing a jumbo syringe full of saline into the tube, down into the stomach; then pulls back on the plunger to refill the emptied syringe with saline and flushed-out stomach contents. After discarding this waste into the basin, she grabs another syringe with fresh saline and repeats the maneuver. Then discards it. Then repeats it again. My job is to examine the discard, to monitor whether pill frag- ments are present. After ten flushes, the effluent from the stom- ach is completely clear. Except for the bloody tinge caused by the tube grating against her stomach lining.

"Looks clear now. Pull it."

The nurse smoothly withdraws the long plastic tube out of the stomach, up the esophagus and out through the mouth. The girl makes a long, deep gasping noise, like a spent diver finally coming to the surface, and vomits one last time into the basin. Vomitus drips from her hair and nose and chin.

"OK. Let's take a break and get cleaned up. Then give the charcoal."

The nurses strip off their protective gear, and begin cleaning up the mess—the used tube, empty syringes, two basins filled with saline and mucus and bloody vomitus, soiled bedsheets and blankets and pillows. Then they clean the girl's face and hair and arms and shaking hands with a washcloth and towel. She blows her nose to clear it. Her gown needs changing. I leave Room B to wash up and change my soiled scrubs.

Time for the binding agent. Liquid charcoal. A thick black gritty liquid slurry. Like drinking wet tar—two large styrofoam cupfuls. It runs through the intestines and binds up and eliminates whatever drug wasn't captured with the lavage. Sipping at the bitter chalky tar is always a slow, distasteful process. The charcoal stains everything it touches black, including lips and teeth. Vampire teeth. It's indelible on clothing. Vomitus and charcoal taught me it's better to work ER in scrubs than streetclothes.

After washing up and changing my scrubs, I re-enter Room B. "How's the charcoal going?"

"We're working at it. Haven't gotten any down yet."

These nurses are showing an extra degree of patience with her. I've known others with little tolerance for this kind of thing. They grumble about having to deal with such "teenager nonsense," especially when the ER is busy with bona fide sick children waiting for care. Some take the irresponsible attitude of "maybe the tube and charcoal will teach them something for the next time." Which ignores the possibility that if the teen makes another "gesture," they might not alert anyone until it's too late because they feared going to the ER.

"What's the problem?" I ask.

"I'm not drinking it," the girl says defiantly.

Time to draw the line. "We don't negotiate the charcoal. It goes down, one way or another. It's your choice—either you drink it, or we have to give it through another tube down the throat. Think it over. I'll be back."

After a few minutes, I return to see the girl is sipping away at the charcoal. I've never had a patient refuse to drink it—all of it—after they hear about the possibility of a second lavage tube.

Her mother has just arrived. She seems embarrassed to be here, like all parents in this difficult situation; it must feel like visiting jail to post bond. A blot on the family name. After introducing myself, I explain what has happened here so far.

After which, I'm never quite sure who to direct myself to in the exam room when there is a teenage patient with their parents. Are teenagers children or adults? Do they want to take responsibility for managing their own health? Most times not. Yet each time I'll show the courtesy and respect of looking at them and telling them what I found, and what tests need to be done; and what treatment is necessary, and why. I look at them and tell them, until they show me they're not much interested in following along. Then check my frustration, and switch the focus onto their parents.

"Do you have any questions about this?" I ask the girl's mother.

"No. You say the blood test will tell if there's a serious problem?"

"Right. Actually, the results should be back by now. I'll go check the computer."

I leave Room B and close the door so they can talk in private. Then log the girl's name into the computer, and strike the key for *Results*—they scroll down the screen: *Acetaminophen level—20mg/dl;* good, far below the toxic range. No need to worry about liver damage. *Urine screen for drugs of abuse—negative. Urine pregnancy test—positive....*

Positive?? No—it can't be. This must be a mistake. *She's only fourteen years old.* I need to confirm this. I call the lab, and ask them to cross-check the patient's name with the results—*yes,* they say, *it's her, it's her urine sample;* and *yes, the test is positive.* I ask them to run it again, hoping there was an error. About fifteen minutes later they call back to say the retest is also positive.

Now what? It's not a routine ingestion case anymore. It's not about school clothes. Who do I give these results to—the girl, or her mother? Both? Should I tell the girl first? Can I tell the mother if I tell the girl first and she doesn't want me to tell her mother? It's her pregnancy. Under usual circumstances, my legal obligation regarding physician disclosure would be to the girl; to respect her right to confidentiality about her health issues if she requests it. *But she tried to commit suicide.* There are more than a few psychological implications attending this case. None of these considerations is mapped out in the protocol I've been following so far.

After mentally sorting through this it makes most sense to tell the mother—first, and in private. Because the girl is only fourteen years old. Psychologically, she's a child; and probably took the pills because she missed her period and suspected she was pregnant. The "gesture" was a cry for help. The fact that she tried to harm herself absolves me of any legal obligation to her right to confidentiality. She needs a support system to get through this; I can't leave it to her to cope alone with this predicament.

Hopefully, her family can be that support. This is no time for name-calling, or accusations, or ultimatums. A teenage pregnancy has deep, long-range implications on many lives; many have to accommodate it, and make compromises: The new mother and father, who lose a big part of their youthful freedoms to decide their futures; the new grandparents, who usually assume the primary responsibility as caretakers of a newborn baby; and the newborn baby, who often grows up in the deficiencies of a less than ideal household. Sometimes it all works out, when everyone rallies to do their best. Rarely. Most times it doesn't, because of all the anger and resentment. . . .

The girl's mother and I are alone, seated across from each other in the Quiet Room. She seems to be awfully tense—agitated, like she can't wait to leave here. Best to give the good news first, about the ingestion being nontoxic; because she probably won't hear anything else after I tell her about the pregnancy test.

"Let me review the test results with you. First of all, the blood test for acetaminophen was far below the danger range, so we don't have to worry about liver damage."

"Oh, that's a huge relief," she exhales. "I was really worried, after you said it could be serious." She starts to rise from her chair. "OK—so, we're all done here now? Can we leave?"

"Well, no. There's more I need to tell you. Have a seat."

We've just hit the steep part of the slope going down. There's no way to ease her into it. No better or worse way to break this kind of news. You have to tell it like the medical fact that it is—then brace for whatever response is offered up, and try to help them cope with the shock.

"We checked a pregnancy test—and it's positive."

"*What? What do you mean?*" she shoots back, with a startled look of pained confusion—as if someone hit her in the face with a pail full of ice-cold water. "Pregnant? I'm not pregnant!"

"No—it's your daughter's test."

"*Who?*"

"Your daughter. Your daughter is pregnant. Which may be why she took the pills—"

"*My daughter? Pregnant? Are you joking?!*" she interrupts, looking angry and panicked, as if ready to lash out at some invisible endangerment closing in on her. Anger, panic, confusion . . . then, strangely, her hardness softened—for just a moment. It seems the human face is incapable of sustaining any pure expression during this kind of shocking confusion; there's always a peculiar mix of many emotions, one overflowing another like fast-moving clouds across a stormy sky. After showing startle, confusion, shock, hurt, anger . . . then

her face softened for just the briefest moment, with a tinge of—
of—*embarrassed glee*. Because every parent hopes to hear these
happy words, imagines it becoming a reality some day—the
news of their child joining in the mystery of bringing new life
into the world. The moment of receiving this wonderful news
is probably rehearsed many times by all parents. And to finally
experience it—even under these jarring circumstances—
caused her an irresistible reflex-spasm of joy. But then all trace
of joy is quickly snuffed out due to its prematurity, and the
hardness of the full reality crept back into her expression.

"I just don't believe it—there must be some mistake," she
protests. "My God—she's just a child."

You have to stick to the unkind facts to keep them focused
when they start to push away reality. I pass her the lab slips
showing the results.

"I ran the test twice to make sure, and it was positive both
times."

"Impossible. *Our family? Pregnant?* How can this happen?"

She seems to want an answer. I don't have one to give. "It's
more common than you might think. The psychiatrist is coming in to evaluate her—maybe he can help answer that."

After a long tense pause, she asks "Now what happens?
What's next?"

"If the psychiatrist finds no suicidal risk, you can take your
daughter home. From a medical standpoint this is considered
a high-risk pregnancy—so I recommend she make an appointment to see an obstetrician."

"An *obstetrician*? She still sees a *pediatrician*. She just started
baby-sitting this summer—so what's a fourteen-year-old girl

supposed to do with *her own* baby? Where can she go in her life after this?"

Then she looked at me, with searching confidential eyes—like so many others before who have sat at this table in this room, negotiating a permanent transition, feeling hurt and lost, needing an answer, and said, "It feels like a part of her died here today." Then asks, "What did I do wrong, doctor?"

I'm the one who's supposed to provide the answers. Yet I'm sure she can tell by the empty look on my face that I don't have one to give for this question, either.

"Would it help if I tell her about it?" I offer.

After another long pause to consider, she says, "Maybe you should. I can't face her now; I wouldn't know what to say. I need to go out and be alone for a while."

Now it's the girl seated across from me. Same room, same table and chairs. She looks preoccupied, almost bored; gazes nonchalantly around the room, won't regard me. And yet the message I bring her today will indelibly stamp her future life forever. Maybe she already suspects what I am about to say—

"Your mom asked me to go over the test results with you. First of all, the blood test for acetaminophen was fine, so there's no risk for liver damage. You should be OK."

She makes no reaction to this news, doesn't look at me or acknowledge what I've just said. Now for the hard part. I can't predict how she'll respond. Will she become hysterical, and run out? Or do something desperate to hurt herself? Or will it be more of this denial? I've seen denial run deep in pregnant teenagers. Just last month an ambulance brought in a full-term newborn baby, just delivered at home—in the toilet—to a teen who claimed she didn't know she was pregnant, even though she gained all that weight and missed her period for eight months. She thought the labor pain was constipation.

"I need to tell you about another test we ran today. Maybe you already know the results. Your pregnancy test—is positive." I don't want this to be ambiguous in any way—*"Which means you are pregnant.* Did you miss your period, and think it was possible? Is that why you took the pills?"

"I didn't take any pills. And I'm sure I'm not pregnant," she mutters, twirling the rings on her fingers.

I pass her the lab slips showing the results. "I ran the test twice—it was positive both times." She makes no reaction, and no movement toward examining the irrelevant papers.

That's it—I've hit the wall with her. There's no penetrating through this depth of teenage denial. I've been here before— it's one of those silent disasters; a quietly thickened morass. When you find yourself waded up to your own neck in it, you just have to let them go.

Is that my pager beeping? I reach down—can't feel it buzzing in my hand. . . . After a moment of this confusion I realize it's not my pager beeping—*it's hers.*

She focuses all her selective youthful energetic concentration like a red-hot laser beam on the pager's digital message, scans every word of it, then looks at me for the first time and says, "That's my friend Sara calling. We're going to the mall today. Can I leave now?"

• • •

After the psychiatrist finished his evaluation, and the discharge papers were signed, I stood at a distance watching the girl getting ready to go. The difficult teenagers always look older to me, after the "gesture" and the experience here that follows. There's a sadness to them, as if they are leaving something irretrievable behind.

As she and her mother walk down the hallway to the exit, I notice the girl is carrying something. Something wrapped in fuzzy brown cloth. Looking more closely, I can make out she is holding a stuffed animal in her hands. A child's toy. And yet earlier in the day those same hands held the balance of her tender life, and had the capacity to tip the scale either way. The same unprepared hands which, in less than nine months, will bear the responsibility for shaping the future welfare of another human being.

There is an ancient myth about a clever man named Daedalus, a great inventor, who made wings of wax to fly and gave them to his son, Icarus. The father cautioned the boy, "Don't go too near the sun. Keep a middle course over the sea." Icarus soared exultantly up and up, and the delight of this new and wonderful power pushed him on even higher, until the wings melted from the heat of the sun above—he crashed into the sea, and the waters closed over him.

Seems I've rediscovered the veracity of this myth more than a few times during my years working ER.

It's always so inspiring to see a young person on the verge of adulthood who is listening and making good decisions.

Other times you see a difficult teenager, a young person with thick shiny hair and a keen eager face set like a springcoil, ready to hatch the kernel of their life, who has brought some abuse onto themselves—an abuse that permanently closes a door to the future. And then all the optimism evaporates with the oasis shimmer of a mirage.

Sometimes you see so clearly into the life of a difficult teenager. Get an eerie, poignant flash of insight into the future when you look deeply into their unmarked face—and see it instantly aged many years. See where the wrinkles will set, how the hair will thin and gray, where will be the scars. Sometimes it urges you to warn them of a present danger in their way— but, like a muted dream of frustration, even though you scream it out, no one seems to hear.

The Discretionary

I recalled the brilliantly lit summer's day sky outside, a high and windless blue, the serene drift of which I got mentally lost in during my ride to the hospital; I drifted back to it again for just a moment, while we pushed full-tilt in the ER resuscitation room—working a code-blue on a little boy. *Daniel.* A three-year-old. Near-drowning victim. Swimming pool at home—he was playing on the patio, next to it; the gate was closed, but not locked. Mom went into the house to turn off the stove, and came right back out . . . he was floating face down in the water, lifeless as a fluttered autumn leaf. She pulled him out and called 911. He was blue and limp, pulseless, not taking breaths. The paramedics administered CPR and rushed him here.

We've been pushing hard to bring him back for two hours now. That's double the usual time recommended for a child presenting in his condition—with no spontaneous heartbeat or respirations, pupils fixed in a fully dilated position, not even an eyeblink movement to him. We did chest compressions, used a machine to breathe him, gave a massive amount of medication to try to stimulate his system. With no response.

Is it time to call it off? Everyone in attendance is weary from pushing back against the oppressive surrounding doom. For two full hours. On final check, the pupils still don't react to light and there are still no palpable pulses. Then, as we silently perform the last remnants of the resuscitation, there comes a noise: Beep . . . beep . . . beep . . . beep. *A heartbeat.* We all hear it beeping, after being transduced by the monitor connected to the wires connected to Daniel's chest. A faint and far too slow beat to sustain him, but at least it's something to build on.

We all looked at each other. *Where did that come from?* After having emotionally acquiesced that this little boy was gone. Then everyone looked at me. *Now what?*

We can't withdraw life support if there's a pulse. If we do— if we stop the chest compressions and mechanical ventilation and IV medications—the faint and slowly beating heart would quickly give out again. For good. So we have to push on. . . .

Someone has to be the discretionary in this situation—to interpret the pattern, make judgments, call out the orders. On the one hand, I feel sure that even if we continued to work our very best at it, even if we retrieved a full heartbeat, the outcome would still be devastation. I feel sure that every precious physical thing vital to this little boy living a normal life has been terribly damaged from all the down-time—brain, heart, kidneys. . . . I can tell when a patient has suffered permanent brain damage by the status of the pupils, the window to the brain.

Daniel's pupils gaped widely, and didn't constrict with the light even after his heart started to beat again; reflecting the dismal status of his oxygen-deprived brain. I feel quite sure that he will never walk, talk, or feed himself; that he'll require continual home-care nursing; that his limbs will stiffen and atrophy, and there will be many hospitalizations and operations and prostheses to compensate the damaged tissues.

On the other hand, I know full well that Daniel's parents are waiting down the hall for some word on their son's condition. . . .

Seems I always scan these conflicting thoughts during the last phase of a futile resuscitation, after reaching a certain point—a point when it's clear there can be no "meaningful" salvage. I weigh them, then ask myself the question—*is it best, to continue trying to bring them back?* I ask because I've seen the aftermath of families with a severely handicapped child—one who suffered the same injury and "came back." Seen the guilt, the bitter accusations, the broken marriages; the effects of attention being displaced from the other siblings, which caused them deep psychological problems later on. I've learned that coming back at all cost isn't always a miraculous thing.

And just as I asked myself the question—*is it best, to continue?*—there came the faint, too-slow heartbeat beeping on the monitor. Only because we had kept at it longer than normal. *How long is "normal"? When do you give up? Or is it more just giving in?* Seems it's different in each case. Research data shows there is little chance for salvage if, after a full hour of resuscitation, the pupils don't react to light and the heartbeat and breathing don't return. Yet research data doesn't take into account the fact that there is a real piece of history—someone's precious child—lying motionless just beneath your hands.

This conflict always contends in my mind and colors my thoughts, sometimes such that one hour on the clock stretches to two. With Daniel, if after the first hour I'd listened in private with my stethoscope to hear the silence within his entombed chest, and shined the light beam again into those glazed eyes with the big dark pupils—seamless eyes, in which you could almost see your own reflection—and *then* had asked myself the question: *Is it right to continue?*—I might have made the judgment to call off the resuscitation, and disconnect the machines.

But I didn't ask myself the question at that point. That was *then*.

The eager heart seems to be beating a little bit faster.

So, what *now*?

Beep . . . beep . . . beep. . . . After resuscitating through the third hour, Daniel's heartbeat is stronger and more regular; he has a sustained pulse and stable blood pressure. We retrieved that part of the working body. Yet he shows no sign of spontaneous activity, his silenced brain tissues are likely lost in the swollen disarray of their anoxia.

With his condition being stabilized for the moment, my next responsibility is to inform the parents. They've surely spent an agonizing three hours sitting in the Quiet Room down the hall—alone, waiting for the doctor to come, waiting for some word. Waiting to hear whether it is a "yes" or "no." There's nothing to do but wait, even though your child is fifty feet away and possibly dying. What do they say to each other?

Sometimes nothing. Sometimes each has to wait alone, even though in the surround of family intimates. There is probably a lot of private deal-making going on in the interim.

The nurses can monitor Daniel in here; they know where to find me if he deteriorates. Just down the hall.

In this business, there's nothing more difficult—no more draining task—than to leave a failed resuscitation to tell parents of their child's demise. The message is horrifying to give, to receive. And then what? Do you conclude with "I'm so sorry"? Is it appropriate to reach out a hand, and touch their shoulder? You are an emissary in this situation, a medium, carrying an irrevocable message that transfers a reality between the two rooms—two worlds. A reality that leaves an indelible mark on everything; because, unlike almost any other eventuality in this life, no adjustment can be made to accommodate it. Nothing—to change the confusion into sensibility, to compensate the loss and suffering by the mental trick of later justifying the experience as being, somehow in the long run, "for the best."

When a child *dies* in the ER I know *what* has to be said to the parents. Even though I never know quite *how* to say it, the message itself is harrowingly straightforward. But what sequence of words strung together can communicate to them that their child's orphaned body survives without the brain? And how should they react to the news? With a sense of relief? Or mourn it like a death? The reality which you must somehow depict supersedes our conceptual boundaries, surpasses any ordinary capacity to grasp, stymies the comfortable faculty of our daily judgment. Conceiving, grasping, judging becomes a *pro-*

cess, which each must somehow come to terms with in their own way.

I paused for a moment in the hallway, just outside the door to the Quiet Room. *How many times have I been here before?* Can never keep my head up, going in. Always feel puny, stripped of all my doctor-authority crossing over this threshold—because there's nothing I can do to stop what's to come.

I paused for another moment, to listen, perhaps to glean something from within that would tell of the situation there. To help anticipate, and prepare myself. I can make out the distinctive deep-staccato rhythm of an angered male voice from inside, but can't decipher what he says. Something tells me that what I have to say—and how I say it—will permanently alter something important between the two strangers inside. Just like so many times before.

I open the door. The parents quickly turn in their chairs to look at me. Two faces rising. Everything stops—is suspended. They don't know me—in this charged situation there's no luxury of introductions; they can't pause to look you over, to take estimate of the messenger, to make the normal judgments of orientation which all parents do in a more "routine" ER situation. It doesn't matter, because they clearly recognized what I represent—*The Word*—I feel it in their turbulent rising-up to hear the message. Their ability to attend is always so utterly focused—to hear the message—because nothing else matters.

It comes blasting like a huge wave. *"Is he?"*—the father's eyes raging and fierce, every muscle in his tensed body set to react. Fury or joy.

"Yes—Daniel is alive . . ." I begin—and yet I know I've done them a necessary disservice as I speak it. Because they leapt to their feet, both of them, and embraced each other with frenzied abandon, wildly screaming—*"Yes, our boy's alive—our son Danny! Oh, God heard our prayers!"* I can't tell who said what, it came out as one last song. They've been unkindly transported to another dimension with a wild savage delirium.

Now I am alone in the room. There is nothing to do but wait for a chance to speak again.

Then the father turns to me, in a shining aura of rapture, and asks, "So, he's going to be all right?"

"We don't know yet," I reply.

Then everything stops again, is suspended in the darkening eye of the storm. Daniel's parents separate, like two exhausted swimmers who realize they are confounding each other, and each has to try for shore on their own.

They stagger bewilderedly back to their chairs.

Father is immediately up again. *This is it—I can tell.* He has that look of absolute contradiction which I've only seen in this situation: Fearlessly panicked, excruciatingly numbed, every which way to go with no way out.

"What do you mean you don't know?" he demands.

What comes next is perpetual solstice, because it will forever taint their future days of restful contentment with the smear and grime and smell of blank mortality.

"The best judgment at this point is that Daniel probably went a long time without oxygen. His exam shows he may have some brain injury."

I can't keep up a full breath through the telling; can't look them in the eye. I describe Daniel's pupils, his overall unresponsiveness, the fact that he's not breathing on his own. Then I explain how a suffocating lack of oxygen to those fragile neural tissues, even for just a few minutes, can cause swelling—like a rubber band wrapped tightly around a finger—and when the brain swells inside the rigid confines of the cranium, the circulation can't pulsate through against the pressure, which can cause permanent damage.

My mouth is awfully dry. *Try to lift up your head.* I make sure they hear me say *possible* risk for brain damage. . . . "We just won't know for at least twenty-four hours. Maybe longer—"

Daniel's father is wild again, all breath and blood, tearlessly sobbing in and out to move his air—

"Brain damage?? After just a few minutes?? Not my boy!!"

I almost can't decipher his words through the guttural sound of his voice. His roaring eyes flash around the room. They brutally light on his wife.

"How long did it take for the paramedics to get to him??" he demanded to know from her.

Daniel's mother did not answer.

"Did you do CPR before they came?!" he shouted ferociously at her.

There is no response; she sits in her chair, blankly staring down at the floor, her arms tightly held across her lap, silently rocking back and forth. Straitjacketed.

"TELL ME! DID YOU DO CPR AFTER YOU PULLED HIM OUT OF THE GODDAMNED POOL??!!" he boomed punishingly with a hoarse, shaking voice.

She looked up at him, with stark vacant eyes, and muttered

something which sounded like "yes." Yet we all knew she probably didn't recall for sure, and that it probably didn't matter.

There is no moment of greater empathy for another human
being than when you see them diminished and suffering due
to loss like that. You just know the black dog's come to stay.
Every facade of individuality is stripped clean away, with Bib-
lical magnitude, as they stand there in stark, naked, pitiful vulnerability. . . . . All because God blinked, or was distracted by
the universe, and turned His back for an instant. . . . Once you
see it, and realize not all suffering is redemptive, it's an elementary thing—elementary—to feel deeply for them; because
when you look at them, and see inside, you find it's really you.

Sometimes I have this dream after a futile resuscitation of a child
on my watch. It's the same dream every time. More like a vivid
remembrance, barely separate from that other world; it almost
feels as if my hand has floated up against the amnion. . . .

*I'm riding an underground train. There is no driver, no
other passengers on board. The doors open at each stop but
no one is waiting to get on. The static on the speaker overhead makes me nervous. I don't have a map, there are no
signs posted outside the window on the tunnel walls, so I
don't know where I'm going; but I do know to keep riding
if I'm to get there. I go for hours it seems, passing the stark
interval glare of naked white bulbs lining the dark tunnel.
How will I know when it's time to stop and get off? Outside
the train I hear the screech of violin strings and whistling*

bats. The wheels ring along the track-grooves like Turkish cymbals, veering whichever way I lean my body. I feel sure of my direction, for the moment—but at some point soon I'll have to decide whether to transfer over. The perspective either way down the track comes to a point. Then the train begins to slow—I'm relieved to finally see commuters crowding the platform. They look disengaged, like pine needles scattered on a forest floor, waiting in long lines like faintly glowing filament. Many are sad, some crying. No one seems to see the train arrive. The doors open, but no one boards. I know this isn't my stop, so I stay on. I feel pity for them, as the hydraulics exhale and the doors close, as the train pulls out and they shrink away behind, passing like combed-out hair rinsed down a sink-bowl drain. . . .

The next day I decided to visit Daniel in the ICU. To get a better sense of what had happened, and of what it all meant.

I entered the quiet hush of his low-lit sickroom. His mother is sitting in a chair at the foot of his bed. Looking down, making notations. Daniel is lying there, motionless—an empire struck down—connected to the monitors, a ventilator machine, the IV pumps; with a catheter in his wrist artery to measure blood pressure and a catheter in his bladder to drain urine into a bag. His legs are covered with a tattered homemade quilt, the bed filled with a regiment of stuffed animals.

I can see she hasn't changed her clothes since yesterday. Or combed her hair. Or slept.

"Hello. I'm the ER doctor from yesterday. Can I come in?"

She looks up. "Why . . . yes," she whispers distractedly. I

can't quite tell through the numbed exhaustion on her face if my presence in the room had really registered.

"I thought I'd stop by before my ER shift. Did you get any sleep last night?"

"Don't think so. Maybe a little."

"It looks like Danny's on a lot of support. How did it go overnight?"

"Well, it was rough there for a while." Then she seemed to lapse into a trance. "His blood pressure dropped about midnight, so we started a medicine called dopamine." She is reading to me from her notes. "In the green bottle hanging there. I had the nurse put different-colored tape on each medicine bottle so I could follow along. The dopamine worked good till—till about 2 A.M., then his pressure dropped again—real low. I got worried, because three doctors came in to work on him. They said his heart muscle might be damaged. We turned up his IV fluids, and added another medicine called *do—dobut—dobutamine*— it's hard to pronounce. Red bottle. Had to go real high with that one to finally get Danny's pressure back up. I keep track of how much urine he makes in the bag every hour, because they said it's a sign of how his heart's pumping; so far so good. No change in the dials on the ventilator machine—his breathing hasn't gotten any worse. The chest x-ray this morning didn't show any pneumonia. I'm thankful for that, because the pool has chlorine and it could've burned his lungs." She scans the next page of her notes. "About an hour ago he had a fever to 104, so we drew more blood to see if there's any infection, and started antibiotics. In the blue bottle. The bottle wrapped in foil has adrenaline, just in case his blood pressure drops again and won't come back up, but so far we haven't had to use it."

With that, she finished on the last page of her notes.

It's always an astonishing thing to witness—the indomitable force generated by the ultimate advocate: A *mother-protectorate*, who has made it her mission to master every aspect of a situation relevant to her stricken child's well-being. There's never any hesitation, never any intimidation. Daniel's mother had stayed at her station all night; I believe she would have steered constellations if it could've opened a door of opportunity—like once before—to another mystical connection, one that would allow her to retransmit the life-force she once gave to her son just three years ago.

"I had the strangest feeling last night, like Danny was still growing inside me; I felt him moving," she muttered, in a distant, private way.

I didn't know what to say to that—it's more like something she said to herself rather than to me. After a bit of silence between us, I ask, "Where's Dad?"

She looked up at me, almost startled—as if it's the first time recognizing my presence in the room. She seemed embarrassed by my asking—to recall my being privy to the horrible confrontation yesterday in the heat of the Quiet Room.

"He had to leave this morning, to take the other kids to school."

"Did you have a chance to talk to any specialists today?"

She shuffled her notes again. "The neurologist was in early this morning, and did some tests. He said Danny's high-risk for having brain damage. But they don't know how much yet."

Then she drifted away from me again. "I think it's too early to tell. I've been talking and singing to him all night, and he blinks his eyes now. He's still our boy. We'll take whatever we get, and do the best we can with it."

You get to a point where there isn't much left to say. Unless you take the conversation onto a more personal level. Which is unnecessary, because you made the visit after your part was done, showed up when you didn't have to. It says enough. After a certain point you are an intruder on a private grief. Yet having nothing more to say in this type of situation isn't the awkward moment it can be in other social encounters—parents consider you to be a friend when you show kindliness toward their child, and an intimate part of the family whenever you go farther. Sometimes sweat is just like blood.

It's time to leave, because my ER shift begins in a few minutes. Daniel's mother is back to sorting her notes. Just before exiting the room, I brush her remorseful shoulder with my hand and wish her good luck, say I will be thinking of them. At the door I turn to look back—to see her sitting there alone, under low lights, tending to what remained of her son's legacy. And for some odd reason, I say to her, "You know, we worked at it longer than normal—to get Danny back."

She looked up at me, distant in her poverty, and nodded; then began sorting her notes again.

After leaving, I felt uncomfortable at having stepped out from behind the mask to say something personal like that. Almost indiscreet. Yet later that day, after working my ER shift and thinking about all the things I wish I'd said during my brief encounters with the families, I hoped it was something she heard and would remember. I don't know where the urge came from to say it—it was one of those spontaneous gestures of fellowship offered to someone caught in deep trouble. The kind of uncalculated gesture you hope can reassure them, in some small way, that despite the tragedy of misfortune there is a connection between people. I had no ulterior motive for saying it, I had nothing to gain; I didn't think I'd ever see her again, so I wasn't seeking her praise or thanks. It was just the truth.

Seems the older I get, the more it feels as if each autumn passing is a personal loss, my own private failing . . . and the harder it is to let go, to give way to the inevitable sweep of the seasons without understanding why.

I remember the autumn that year stretched deep into October. The trees changed their essence late. They were especially beautiful in the rain—the dark wet bark, the umbrellate branches, their cold enameled leaves—like colored buoys on a clanging tide. . . . Then came the first night of hard frost, and the next day it seemed the big linden in the front yard went underground; it was stripped barren in just one afternoon.

On the last day of autumn it snowed. A hard, blowing snow. Hood up, head down, I made white tracks going out on the trail. They were almost covered over on my way back. There was a hand-addressed envelope in the mailbox; inside, a large color photograph of Daniel—strapped into his wheelchair, connected to a ventilator machine and cardiac monitor. His spastic arms and legs already appeared to be a bit spindly and twisted. There was no expression on his deeply damaged face;

he sat upright, full-lit by the waning sun, surrounded by the hugs and valiant smiles of his mother and brother and sister.

Then I turned over the photograph, and read the simple, handwritten inscription on the back, which said, "*Thank you for giving us our son Danny back.*"

Hands Washing

JUNE 4, 1996

6 A.M.–10 P.M.

BEFORE THE OVERNIGHT SHIFT

6 A.M. Exactly. I always know what day it is when I automatically wake at exactly 6 A.M. without a prompt from the alarm clock, and when I feel this peculiar anxiety drumming inside. It means I'm working the overnight shift in the ER tonight. I wake early, and feel anxious, because there is a lot to do to get ready before going in.

The ER overnight shift. I've certainly worked my share of them through the years. Usually one per week. It seems you never forget the nocturnal contradiction. Let me try to describe the phenomenon: Simply put, I go in to the ER at 10 P.M. tonight, work there all night long, then go home at 9 A.M. the next morning. Simply put.

Yet it's more than just an eleven-hour ER shift; more like a thirty-six-hour cycle of physical and mental inversion. Because to work the overnight tonight, I have to wrench my body out of its comfortable diurnal rhythm, and push it—to nap this afternoon *before* the shift, then stay awake all night to work my best *during* the shift, then go home tomorrow morning and force myself to nap (fitfully) for a few hours *after* the shift. Then, waking unrested sometime early tomorrow afternoon, limp in first gear through what's left of the day, then retire to bed tomorrow evening for a "full" night of sleep. Without any residue of physiologic perplexity.

I discovered early in my ER career that the body wasn't made to go inside out like this. It hurts each time; and takes at least two days to recover from. So there has to be some justification made for continuing to work the overnights. I rationalize it as a necessity, since the ER is open twenty-four hours a day, and serves as an after-hours private-practice office for the entire city. The overnights are part of the job working ER. I justify it driving in to work them, and again driving home the next morning.

An ER doctor never forgets his worst overnight shifts. Those in which there is literally no time—to eat, or rest, or even use the lavatory—for eleven straight hours. Humorless nights spent running from room to room, patient to patient—overwhelmed with business, with no time to collect yourself; not even for a moment just to wash your face.

Why is it so difficult?

One reason is you work alone. On other ER shifts you share the workload with another doctor. But on overnights it's just you managing the entire unit and whatever load of patients presents during the night. Some nights they come rushing in waves—sick children, with vomiting and diarrhea, pneumonia, croup, meningitis, dehydration, asthma ... and there is no doctor-partner to help pick up the slack. So you have to spread yourself as thinly as possible to keep it all going—examining patients, discussing your findings with their parents, writing orders, performing technical procedures like IVs and spinal taps and stitching cuts, interpreting lab tests and inspecting x-rays; then re-examining the patients, discussing a management plan with their parents, making phone calls to update their private pediatricians, writing prescriptions and discharge instructions. . . . Somewhat like an acrobat on a TV variety show, running from stick to stick trying to keep all the plates spinning on top. Sometimes it feels like you are barely treading water, and have to spread yourself so thin to keep it all going that it comes close to creating a dangerous situation.

Another reason is the physical discomfort that gnaws inside you during the night. From being tired and hungry. You can't do anything about the "tired" component—so you eat. No matter how busy, you have to make time to eat something, especially once your hands start to shake from all the caffeine. But eating never satisfies on an overnight shift, because of the distraction of thinking and doing and worrying about what comes next. And you have to be so careful about what you eat—because if you eat too much food out of frustration, or the wrong kind of food out of convenience (like red meat with gravy from the cafeteria, or a load of candy from the vending machine), you become light-headed from digestion, and have trouble concentrating. *So, just how much tuna fish and hard boiled egg-white can one hungry doctor eat during an eleven-hour shift? How many bananas?* And then there's the nausea to contend with the next day, from all the coffee it took to trick the gears of your body to finish. . . .

Another reason is the predictable waning of your concentration. There is only so much of it to stretch through the night; it becomes more and more difficult to focus as the shift wears on. Sometimes you look at an x-ray, and look and look again, and still can't make sense of what you see. As if the connections are loose. Sometimes when ordering a dose of medication you do the same calculation over and over and get a different value each time. There are high stakes involved, because too much sodium in the IV bag and the patient could have a convulsion, or not enough sodium in the IV bag and the patient could have a convulsion. It's especially sobering to be responsible for calculating a dose of chemotherapy for a child with cancer, when an error in the placement of a decimal point can result in a lethal dose being given. Once you fail at basic math, it's time to regroup—leave the ER, even for just a few minutes, to try to shake it off. I usually go to my office and close the door, and look out the window deep into the murmur and hum of the twinkling universe. Sometimes looking out makes me wonder about other people, how they live and work, and what they are doing with their lives. After a few minutes of looking and wondering, it's time to go back.

Working the overnight shift becomes more difficult over the years. They tug at you with a grounding inertia that wobbles the smooth spin of your career. So in order to achieve any degree of longevity in the field you must somehow, some way, come to terms with them—try to understand their dynamics, find ways to cope, use tricks to affect their outcome to your advantage. You must either make peace with them, or else practice in a different subspecialty—because overnights are bigger than you; they will be what they will be. And if you can't find a way to negotiate working them, you can expect a big chunk of your ER shift-work to be soured by frustration. . . .

Most people think you just change clothes and go in. Not so. Take today, for instance: I've spent most of it preparing for my overnight shift. All ER doctors use a routine to prepare, which they stubbornly cling to out of insecurity. The routine is the only thing within your control to help you cope with it.

What exactly constitutes the "best" routine is a hotly debated issue among practitioners in the field. *How long do you nap before? Do you exercise? What do you eat? Do you park your car in the same lucky spot each time?* The younger ER doctors want to know, so as to gain longevity in the field. The older doctors, who quit ER after being worn down by overnights, usually grumble some bitter sentiment about how "the only good routine is a day job with regular hours." It seems there's no consensus, probably because there are as many self-indulgent coping strategies as there are idiosyncratic doctors using them.

Today I went through my own routine. Because it makes me feel good, physically and mentally. Since each of these eleven-hour shifts is eleven hours of mostly denying your self, your personal wants and needs, I compensate by making it feel like I took care of myself before going in.

I got up early, at 6 A.M., and spent the first few hours sipping coffee and working on research at the computer. When the sun was up, I went out to do yardwork—raking, sweeping, gardening—any kind of rhythmic physical activity and breathing the fresh air, which is well suited to quiet thinking. At noon, I ate a bagel and some fruit—always something light; but never *after* noon, because then I'll still be digesting later in the day when I go jogging. After eating, I napped for a few hours; then got up, and had another cup of coffee. Back in college, I found that a cup of coffee after a nap resharpened my concentration after sitting through a full day of classes, and allowed me to focus on my studies deep into the night. Those few hours I spent napping earlier this afternoon is all the sleep I'll get during the next twenty-hour stretch.

Late in the afternoon I jogged a quiet seven-mile course of country roads along the river. The route is secluded, so it's rare to encounter another runner. There are wonderful things to see and feel along the way: The euclidean pattern of hawks grazing the summer sky after a fresh wheat cut; the magnificent August cornfields fanning the humid afternoons, so full and lush-green they simmer blue heat; the late autumn soy crop dried to a crisp yellow ocher, when the crickets sing all day and deer begin to scent panic in the fields. It's especially quiet running alongside the river; sometimes the only sound is the ver-mouthed gliding of the water's current just beyond, or the drone of a propellered plane as it passes far above. . . . Today I finished my run at dusk, at the cusp of the day, and watched the sun setting on the horizon—illuminating the upper skies with that special softened glow, a mixture of yellow and orange and red, the kind of transition that urges a sailor home.

I always see more clearly, and remember more fully, jogging

on a day leading up to an overnight shift. The private rhythmicity of breathing and pulsations is almost hypnotic; it opens
channels of thought penetrating far beyond what is practical.
An hour of hard exercise recharges with a bonus energy which
lasts far into an overnight shift; I can feel it helping when I
need that extra gear to get through it. I always finish running
the full seven-mile course no matter what the weather or how
tired I feel near the end, because if I quit early on my jog, I
might be tempted to quit early in some way on my shift.

So—to prepare for tonight's overnight shift, I woke early
and had my coffee and worked at the computer, then worked
in the yard; then ate, napped, had more coffee, and took an
hour of exercise. Nothing else works as well for me, because
after all this, I feel my best—like I have taken care of myself a
little. Years of living with a routine conditions you to automatically measure out life in hourly intervals: Eleven working
makes an overnight shift, two napping hones your concentration, one running covers about seven miles of country road . . .
and one hour spent resuscitating a child without regaining a
pulse is an inexplicable loss.

Living with a routine helps you cope. Yet an ER doctor never
resolves the dread anxiety of being overwhelmed with chaos
deep in trenches of overnight duty—working alone at high
stakes, spreading yourself as thinly as possible without creating
a dangerous situation, being hungry and tired and nauseated,
your concentration waning. The best you can do is accommodate it as a thievish cycle in your life. And accommodate
the permanent change inside—the personal blemish—once

you realize that even during your time off there is always a part of you on alert, forever in a triage mode, conditioned to anticipate and prepare for and react to what comes next.

9 P.M. It's time now, to go in. It's soothing to be insulated in the cocoon of a commute to work, to wind up before a shift and to wind down after. A commute can be anything you want it to be. It's usually private time spent thinking about things, rummaging through the personal compartments of your life. Taking inventory, reaffirming everything is quite all right on that particular day—your family, your health, the direction of your career, finances, future goals. . . .

Sometimes I'll think about what it takes to do the ER job well, by reviewing how I managed a difficult case on the last shift, critiquing how it all went and considering whether I could have done better. Or I'll rehearse a certain scenario, like a resuscitation, to make certain I recall drug doses and where all the equipment is in the room—should it happen that night. Reviewing and critiquing and rehearsing can help you to prepare and anticipate—to strategize, react and determine the next best move. Like an urgent game of chess. Sometimes on a commute I'll remind myself to be patient with the parents, even if they come in with a trivial problem at 3 A.M. *Don't forget*— no one who comes to the ER wants to be there; they come fearing their child is in trouble, and the only thing worse is to leave thinking that no one there listened.

During tonight's commute I thought about what I bring to the job—how each time I try to do my best, and how each time my best seems to get a little better. And it occurred to me, again, that there comes a time in every life when you get the opportunity to push yourself, to see how far you can go; a time to remember much later, after all the struggling, to relish the fleeting interval when you were young and strong and tried your best and did good work. *It's supposed to be hard.* Then I recalled a case in which what I did made a difference—when someone who was downed recovered, in the best way allowable by physiology and fate—because of me, my knowledge and skills, the choices I made for them.

It's good to recall something you did that made a difference in this life. Even once. It's especially good to recall it during a commute to the ER to work an overnight shift. . . .

After the deserted freeway and the exit ramp and the dark downtown streets, I enter the underground parking lot of the hospital. The day-shift workers have long gone home. Then walk through the empty basement tunnel and up the back staircase one flight, then down the hallway over to my office. It's a quiet private walk under the hum of fluorescent lights, a last opportunity to collect myself before beginning the shift. I almost never encounter anyone if I come in this way. Just around the corner from my office is the ER. The invisible pattern of noisy chatter there among the staff tells how busy it is, and can predict what kind of night it will be. One group conversation with relaxed laughter means it's been a slow night; whereas many separate and quick-paced conversations, or no conversation at all, usually means it's busy and will likely stay that way.

Once inside my office, I close the door and change into

scrubs, clip my ID badge onto my shirt, and put the laminated reference card listing drug doses in my breast pocket. Comes in handy at a glance during the panic of a resuscitation, when sometimes I can't even recall the correct spelling of my own name. Everyone needs a pocket card, no matter what their level of experience. Then I hang my stethoscope around my neck— the only one I've ever owned, the one used to listen to the hearts and lungs of every patient I've ever cared for.

I quickly sort through the mail that has accumulated since last shift. Just before going out, I sit for the last quiet moment I'll know for the next eleven hours, to finish accepting what is to come.

9:59 P.M. It's time to lift up, and go out to the ER. Each overnight shift is a contest against yourself, an eleven-hour personal struggle against natural urges: The urge to give out when you are tired and hungry, give up when you are frustrated with too much chaos being thrown at you, give in and cut corners when you are spread too thinly working alone. You see your face reflected in the rear-view mirror on the commute home the next morning; it's a good commute if you can say you overcame those urges and won a small personal victory over yourself keeping the watch.

It's time. I always enter the ER through a doorway to the back room where the nurses take their dinner break, and start with a half-cup of hot coffee. But only a half-cup, because a full cup of caffeine on an empty stomach after jogging seven miles will cause my hands to tremor at the beginning of the shift. You never know when the first task of the evening will be to stitch a cut on a child's face. After the coffee, I glance out into the ER arena to count the number of charts of new patients waiting to be seen, and to see which doctors I will be relieving from the evening shift. That bit of orientation being done, it's time to enter the noise and the glare of the overnight shift.

10:01 P.M. The clock always moves forward. I always take a new pen from the plastic bin on the counter. My only fetish working ER is to use a new pen to write with each shift. Then clean the plastic diaphragm on the head of my stethoscope with an alcohol pad. Then wash my hands with the brown iodine soap from the dispenser over the sink. Sometimes I look at my hands washing and think of all the children they've examined, and I can feel a continuity in all the years that came before— and then they look so strong and capable. . . . Then I pick up the chart of the next patient waiting to be seen. . . .

A Private Shining

JUNE 4, 1996
THE EMERGENCY ROOM
CHILDREN'S HOSPITAL

Excuse me, Doctor, but as soon as you finish in here, we need you in Room Ten."

The nurse requesting this is standing in the doorway, as I place the last stitch in the lacerated chin of a young boy. Raymond. Struck it on a tabletop, split it open. Cut deep, down to the jawbone. Bled all over the front of his shirt. Bruised, but not fractured.

Raymond panicked when he heard the word "stitches." It took a lot to calm him; I explained there would be no shots—that I would numb the cut by coating it with Novocain gel, then he wouldn't feel the stitches. He has apprehensively trusted me, and so far my word is good. The experience has been smooth and pleasant for him and his parents.

Until now. The nurse in the doorway has a formal, pressed tone to her voice; a signal to me that something is wrong. There is no actual "Room Ten" in our ER. "Room Ten" is a code word—for an "utmost-urgent case" coming by ambulance.

"I'm finishing the last stitch now," I say, without looking up.

"OK. We're getting set up for it."

"Good. Be right there."

My tone is likewise formal, which feels awkward since I'm speaking to someone I have worked with for years. Yet it communicates a mutual understanding of the seriousness of her request without alarming Raymond and his parents.

One more stitch to go. I have to shift gears—focus my hands on finishing quickly, yet carefully—symmetrically, the needle-in needle-out at the same depth on each side of the cut, dab away the scant blood pooling with gauze; *don't rush it,* tie the square knot with a proper degree of tension so the wound edges are approximated—just so. Yet my mind has already raced ahead into "Room Ten." *What will it be? Severe head trauma? Cardiac arrest? A gunshot wound? And how will I manage it?*

I have to pull myself back, to concentrate on tying this last square knot. Without actually looking, I can tell that Raymond's parents are studying my face—and from the new quiet between us, they seem to sense something is wrong just down the hall. Seems the parents of an ill or injured child quickly develop an astute empathy for another family's medical predicament. I avoid their eyes, so as to appear to be single-purposed, to maintain their confidence that I will finish the task at hand. Even though mentally I've transferred my concern onto the next case.

Finished. Looks good. I cut the tails of the last stitch close to the knot, then switch on my automatic voice.

"All done now. A nurse will be in to bandage the cut and give you instructions on how to take care of it." I'm edging toward the door. "Your private doctor can take the stitches out in the office next week. It came together nicely, should heal well."

I've said this a thousand times over the years; I scan their faces to determine if it was enough. They nod approval, their eyes seem to convey a silent thank you. But there is nothing actually said; they ask no questions, they seem to understand that I'm pressed for time.

I peel off my bloody rubber gloves inside out into the wastebasket and slip into the hallway, just as the paramedics wheel an empty stretcher past me, heading back in the direction of the ambulance bay. Looking the opposite way, I spot two nurses scurrying about the bed in a room down the hall, hovering with two other anxious adults.

That's where it is. My gait automatically quickens in that direction, hurries, but without running. I've learned to never run. Everyone else can run, but not the doctor. Because these parents will immediately scrutinize me when I enter their lives—lives now forced by a turn of events to seek the aid of strangers, strangers now privy to the inner mechanism of a family crisis—a family crisis involving the well-being of its most precious commodity.

I walk to the bedside and look. There is a tiny newborn baby girl lying there, at most only a few days old; she's having an epileptic convulsion—her eyes blankly staring, vacant of sensation, their gaze deviated to the right, her left arm jerking, fluttering eyelids, saliva bubbling from her mouth.

There are few conditions more frightening to parents than a convulsion. It explodes a repetitive burst of electrical intensity through the corridors of the brain, then gathers and washes down like a cataract over the entire body—the undercurrent taking grip, wrenching every affected muscle in tonic-clonic spasm—and when it resolves, leaves an exhausted consciousness in its wake.

The brain is like an intricate circuit board, finely coordinating the passage of a multitude of signals along neural wires. When the circuitry is overloaded by the electrical firestorm of a convulsion, there is only one gross signal—repetitive, garbled, incoherent. No wonder in times past these "seizures" were thought to be caused by demonic possession—the mentation completely blanked out, the body violently contorted and manipulated by some dark invisible force.

This is serious—critical—because a convulsion in a newborn baby can cause brain damage if it persists too long. How long is too long? No one knows exactly, but it's always assumed that every minute counts. My job here is to preserve every bit of her neurologic capacity, the tender newness of which is so susceptible to damage from this kind of stress. This little baby girl is in the vicegrip of a convulsion, with no sign of breaking free—

I make eye contact with the parents, and introduce myself. "What's her name?" I glance back and forth between them.

"Grace," the father nervously blurts out.

"When did this start?" Hearing a voice, and enabling them to speak to it, usually helps to calm them a bit. And helps me to identify the decision-maker by who answers first.

"About an hour ago," his voice quivers back, as he struggles to maintain control. "Maybe longer. It's been on and off since then. I don't understand—the birth was normal, everything was fine at the hospital afterward. What do you think is wrong?"

This isn't the best time to say. Because they could panic if I tell them it's an epileptic convulsion without a full explanation of exactly what that is. And then I'll have *two* big problems to manage—the baby, and her parents. There just isn't time for a detailed explanation right now, because starting treatment for the baby comes first. Yet if I seem to be evasive they might question my capability, or worry that I'm concealing something of grave importance to spare them. You have to feel for the right time.

The father is fearful, struggling for control, yet seems rational and isn't interfering. I need to maintain that. The mother is teary, quietly agitated, anxious; she seems to be leaning on her husband to negotiate this.

I've seen enough here for my resuscitation mode to click on. The professional part of my brain is spinning its revolving file . . . spinning, until it lights on the invisible mental card with the information I need to manage this case—marked "Newborn Convulsion." I quickly scan the entry; then tell the nurses, "Let's give some oxygen."

It seems an unspoken boundary is crossed, once the doctor gives an order directing care in a critical case like this—and you can feel the parents' willingness to give over their control as caretakers, give it over to you with an almost religious sense of belief.

Convulsion begets convulsion, so the longer it persists, the more difficult it is to quell; and the greater the risk for brain injury. Prioritizing is the key here; to anticipate and stay ahead of what I see in front of me, which is the best way to prevent complications.

Check the patient's vital signs. Fortunately, they are stable at this point. But that could change quickly, and must be monitored very closely.

I need to engage the parents again, to maneuver them away from the bed so we can work without interference. My voice automatically modulates to sound confident, calm and controlled, directed—yet without the inflection that would invite any further questions, because there just isn't time for that now.

Be direct with them—

"It looks like Grace is having a convulsion. Which means that a spot in her brain is over-firing signals."

Be positive—

"Her vital signs are stable, which is the most important thing right now."

Give them direction—

"So we need to start an IV and give her medication to stop it, then run some tests to find out why this happened. I'll try to let you know what we're doing as we go, but we need to get started. OK?"

"Yes, Doctor, OK, do what you have to," the father acquiesces.

The mother is looking down; she is trembling, crying harder now, holding her baby's stilled hand, probably wondering if this will be the last time.

Give her a moment.

"Grace is my first baby. We just went home from the nursery, and everything was going fine. I just fed her an hour ago. How can she be so sick now? Is she going to have to stay in the hospital?"

One of the nurses explains why the answer to the last question is "yes" as she leads them over to chairs in the corner of the room.

We need to get moving on this. I turn to the nurses. "I'm going to start an IV and draw blood for the usual lab tests. If she's still seizing after that, we'll give medication."

The actual sequencing of this is effortless. It clicks into place as if I'm reading it off my invisible mental card. I'm confident it is the right card and has all the information I need.

This confidence in managing a difficult case is what all doctors work to attain their entire career. It comes only after many years of managing many cases, of struggling through them in all their different permutations. Then one day it seems the tumblers click into place—a door opens, and you see the job with a new clarity. It's a mysterious thing, intuitive—like gaining the gift of an extra faculty which can instantly transform the few facts before you into a clear mental blueprint showing the best possible route for proceeding.

A clear mental blueprint: *Newborn Convulsion: Give oxygen→ check the vital signs → start an IV → draw the blood tests → give the anticonvulsant medication. . . .* One-two-three linear thinking. Seeing the best route clearly laid out helps to remove the fear of managing a critical case—the fear of being caught deep in the midst of it and losing your way, and then freezing up and going blank and causing a bad outcome. It gives a confidence that you can make good decisions to effect the best possible outcome, even though the heavy weight of doom is palpably pressing on someone lying just beneath your hands.

This confidence isn't complacency—no. Because you still have to drive each encounter, judge each option along the route and make the right decisions on how best to proceed. So your nerves are charged up with each critical case, because each time driving is a test of your seamanship in some unique way. Yet being charged up with nerves doesn't confound you or block you from doing your best, like fear can. Nerves without fear is good—it engages you to the task, focuses your concentration in a way like nothing else can.

Focus.

I check the start time on the clock—2 A.M. *Don't forget to recheck it often.* Sometimes the clock is your only link to reality after moving deep into the warp of a resuscitation.

The convulsion has been ongoing now for five minutes. Longer, if we add the time at home. We need to give an anticonvulsant medication to stop it. Through an IV line—literally a lifeline—by inserting a thin, one-inch-long plastic catheter tube into a vein. Any vein will do; the sooner the better. Placing an IV in a newborn baby is not an easy task; the veins are tiny, some as small as hollowed-out thread, with tissue paper-thin walls. Difficult to see. Impossible to feel under the skin.

A quick inspection of her blurred, convulsing body shows only one visible vein—in the scalp. I've had parents panic with scalp IVs; one father actually grabbed my hand to stop me, for fear that needling the scalp would in itself cause brain injury. There's no time to walk over and explain this decision to these parents, because the baby's seizure is intensifying. Yet I have to keep alert to their reaction.

The nurse helping me has a difficult job—securing the oxygen mask over the baby's face while holding the head and body steady for the IV try; all during the rhythmic shaking of the seizure. Although it takes firm hand pressure to do so, she must appear to be gentle for the parents' sake.

Prioritize. First, the tourniquet—a thin rubber band placed tightly around the lower scalp like a headband. Then a quick alcohol scrub of the skin overlying the vein. I pierce the tiny IV catheter tip just a few millimeters beneath the skin, with the stealth of a mosquito. Now the delicate part—probing the unseen tissues beneath with the sharp action-end of the catheter tip, at an angle and depth which usually works for me, hoping to engage the vein wall and enter its hollow. Probing, hoping. I'll know that I'm in when I see blood flash back into the hub part of the catheter—

Millimeters seem like miles. If I probe too vigorously, I'll cut all the way through the tiny vein; then it will bleed under the skin and can't be used. *Don't forget—it's the only one.* A flashback of blood indicates that I'm in. *Probe for it carefully.* I can barely see the thin blue line of the vein now. So difficult—

to keep the catheter on a straightward advance with the rhythmic seizing motion. Like blindly threading the roving eye of a small needle.

I advance the tip further—millimeter by millimeter—just beneath the tender, almost transparent newborn skin, to contact that blood vessel I saw more distinctly before placing the tourniquet, watching the hub of the IV for a flashback of corpuscular red, glancing down to check the baby's breathing, one ear to the parents watching our performance. *What time is it now? No—check it later—don't take your eye off that vein.* The parents always seem to focus on my hands and face in these critical situations, so I have to keep both steady.

I should be into the vein at this depth. Yet no flashback. Where is it? Am I off to one side? Or too deep? *Don't rush.* Better to pull the catheter back a bit, then redirect. *What if I can't get this IV in her?* Negative thoughts like that always seem to creep in during the middle of a critical case; they can interfere, make everything harder. So you learn ways to block them out. Last time it was the Gettysburg Address; tonight. . . .

I change the angle of the catheter, ever so slightly; then advance it just another half-millimeter . . . now I feel just the slightest "pop"—almost a "give" sensation—transmitted along the catheter to my fingers. It's more the *absence* of something than the presence of something; a minuscule decrease in resistance, which takes years of performing this procedure to appreciate because of its subtlety. It signals that the catheter tip has just pierced through one side of the vein and is into the hollow. I can't feel this sensation through rubber gloves, so I don't wear them anymore. This time I feel it—it's the same welcomed tactile sensation as all the other times, only modified a bit, because my brain had to subtract out the baby's seizing motion from my fingertips.

The catheter should be in. I need confirmation—hold for a moment—*OK!* There it is, the slow purpled reflux of blood into the hub. Hands keep steady; it's still possible, yet would be unforgivable, to do something mechanically inept to lose it now.

It's not in until it's all the way in. Now to thread the full length of the catheter into the tiny vein. I shift my hands ever so slightly, to stabilize it in place—right there, just at that angle and depth; then pull a slight degree of back-tension on the skin for traction, then gingerly thread the tiny plastic catheter. It slides in with victorious fluidity. Luckily it didn't bend or kink.

You learn the hard way that no one else handles the IV until it's completely secured and you are ready to give it over. I tape the outside part firmly to the scalp, draw a blood sample through it into an empty syringe, then flush it with saline solution, which passes into the vein without resistance.

All is well with this. We've secured access. Now the nurse can connect the IV to the tubing and pump.

Now check the time—2:22 A.M. It took twenty-two minutes to get the IV in. Twenty-two minutes. I've done better; but I should be thankful that it's in. We are part way there. Another quick check of Grace's breathing—it's good so far, surprisingly good. Her chest rises and falls with regularity, there is full air entry into her lungs when I listen with the stethoscope. Her skin is still pink. But the convulsion is escalating—now *both* arms and legs are twitching, her tiny white fists are clenched

166 ◆ William Bonadio, M.D.

tight. This little baby is being shaken by a dark invisible force. She's fighting it with everything she has. But if it spreads any further it will overwhelm her chest muscles and confound air movement—then comes risk of brain damage.

I can see the parents in my peripheral vision. They sit helplessly, forced to occupy those hectic chairs and watch us from the corner. Anonymously, like so many others before, hoping the large warm hand of strength will reach down to touch their child. My body language is the only communication I can afford them. Whether I feel it or not, I have to appear to be unafraid; controlled, confident, directed. This will tell for now.

Now to quell the convulsion. Big decision. There are many anticonvulsant medications to choose from; each has benefits and risks when given to a newborn baby. My mental file spins to the card marked "Valium" to weigh this intervention. Valium is a good choice, because it works quickly—in minutes. Other medications take longer. Time is against us. Valium causes sedation—which is desirable, because it will quell the convulsion; yet undesirable, because it will depress her drive to breathe. We lose precious ground if she stops breathing, because then I'll have to perform the risky procedure of placing a breathing tube into her windpipe to respire her with a machine.

No question we need to quickly snuff out this escalating convulsion, because with each passing moment there's an immeasurable stress weighing on this baby's brain. But Valium is a more appropriate anticonvulsant for older children and adults. I can't recall ever giving it to a newborn—its effects are unpredictable, it could depress her respirations to the point where she'll need the breathing tube. Placing a breathing tube, which is the size and shape of a curved drinking straw, through the tiny mouth down the throat and into the tiny windpipe deep within the unlit confines of her twitching body—at 2:24 A.M., when I am tired and tense with nerves, and there is no one else in the hospital to call for backup if I can't get it in—with the nurses and parents watching—knowing that if I fail the baby could suffocate and die while in my hands, all because of an intervention I chose—

I had luck with the IV. But placing a breathing tube can be much more difficult—it's a blind shot; most times your hands shake; sometimes you just can't find the tiny opening to that tiny windpipe. The patient isn't breathing during your struggle to get the tube in; the books teach you to hold your own breath while attempting to place it, so you can tell how long they've been without oxygen. Most times it's less than a minute before you feel the tingling panic of your own suffocation coming on.

Valium—yes, or no? Hippocrates taught *"primum non nocere,"* which means "first, do no harm." Don't make things worse by your intervention. He also taught that "desperate conditions require the most desperate remedies." The Greeks are no help to me now. Nor are any of my textbooks.

You must always do these deliberations silently in your head. If you think them out loud, you will appear to be unsure of which direction to take—and the nurses and parents will lose confidence.

I finish scanning my mental card on "Valium" several times, so I'm sure I've considered everything there is and can justify the logic of my decision. Top priority is to quell the convulsion—*now*. Sometimes you have to seed a small fire to quench a larger one.

"Let's give Valium."

The nurse passes me the syringe containing the medication. It looks like a clear oil held up to the light, with wavy fluid lines distorting the numbers and gradations printed on the cylinder. Once hand-pumped into the IV tubing, it will be rapidly machine-pumped through the IV tubing, then into the catheter and then into the vein; then be heart-pumped through the bloodstream and diffuse like ether through the cerebral portals, bathing the neural tissues, suffusing beneficial effect like spring rain, calming the electrical firestorm.

Check the time—2:25 A.M. Grace has been seizing for thirty minutes. Only thirty minutes ago I expected to have it stopped by now. *Go.* I insert the syringe tip into a port on the IV tubing, and slowly push the plunger. All of the medication is in. I can see it moving through the plastic tubing, the wavy oil-bolus interposed in the water solution like a bubble in a carpenter's level, pulsing steadily forward toward the vein like a magic bullet clicked into the chamber ready for discharge. Then it disappears into the baby's circulation.

Now we must all hold tight, stare at the convulsing baby, wait for the effect. Deduce the tide-pull by the direction and pitch of the waves. . . . Monitor Grace's convulsion—breathing—vital signs, monitor my body language, monitor the parents' reaction. I've already spun my mental file to the card marked "Breathing Tube," and will hold it in clear view, just in case. All the equipment is set up, if I need it. . . . What

I need is just enough juice to stop the convulsion, but not enough to stop her drive to breathe. . . .

The sweep-hand of the clock has circuited several minutes after giving the Valium to Grace. It should have worked by now. Yet still no change. *Do I need to give more?* I don't want to risk giving another dose because it will surely stop her breathing—

And then there seems to be something different in the over all pattern—as if something invisible is pushing back. Because the baby's convulsion is slowing, its rhythmicity is breaking up a bit, becoming intermittent. The medication has apparently reached its grip onto the proper valve and is turning it clockwise, choking it to a drip. Then, after another minute or so, the convulsion is completely snuffed out.

What a relief.

Don't be relieved. Because now there is hardly any movement to her—she's gone completely limp. Stay on top of it—this is a crucial phase to get through, to ascertain and correct the overshoot. Is she still breathing? Close inspection shows the tiny bellows of her chest is still moving up and down—but it is irregular, diminished . . . yet not stopped. Part of the price.

I have the breathing tube in hand—*hold back*—don't jump at it too quickly, she's still fighting with us; try to work with the effort she has. If I can keep her stimulated, even for just the next few minutes, even by pinching her toe, the painful sensation can now make way to her consciousness—and her cry will pull in and push out deeper breaths until the breathing drive resets at this lower sedated level. Breathing begets breathing. I don't want to cause Grace any more pain, she's already known too much of it during her short time here. But this is the most benign way to avoid having to place the tube—

Each interval pinch of her tiny toe brings a purposeful withdrawal of her leg—a grimace—a brief cry, and with it a welcomed deep breath, indicating an awakening consciousness. After several minutes of this, Grace is sustaining her own vigorous respiratory effort. The convulsion is ended.

2:32 A.M.

For the first time in over a half-hour I can fully straighten myself upright. And can feel the painful cramp stinging in my neck and back. It's safe to move away from the bedside, make way over to the frightened parents and give them a report on what has happened and what we did and what it all might mean.

"Grace is doing well now. Resting quietly. We got the convulsion stopped with the medication. The most important things, like her breathing and blood pressure, were stable the whole time. She'll be transferred from here to the ICU, where they can monitor her very closely. Specialists will be in later this morning to do some tests to figure out why this happened. But for now she's doing OK. Do you have any questions for me?"

They don't. They seem to be relieved, yet bewildered and exhausted. And are either unaware that bad news could follow in the days ahead—or are fully aware, but need a break from all this. It would be almost cruel to burden them with any more speculation at this time. And fruitless, since they seem to be incapable of processing that type of information just now. It is best done in steps. Let them have their new daughter back.

Grace is transferred from the ER to ICU. Her condition is listed as "stable." I wish her parents good luck as they leave our unit; they nod acknowledgement, their eyes seem to convey a silent thank you. Then I wash my hands with the brown iodine soap from the dispenser over the sink. Sometimes I look at my hands washing. . . .

A philosopher once wrote, "But do your work, and I shall know you." You come to realize over the years working ER that your name is seldom remembered after your part is done, and that it's rare to hear if what you did ultimately made a difference. I don't know what ever happened to Grace after our difficult overnight encounter. I *do* know that we received her in critical condition, made decisions and intervened, and then she left our unit stabilized, with her parents.

That's the reality of it. Even though sometimes you need more, it's often all you get; and in that morsel of certainty, you must learn to savor a confidential feast of personal satisfaction. It's a private shining.

Is it enough to keep you going? Maybe not. Maybe so: Once you come to accept that a profound part of any doctor's work is spent toiling in anonymity. And, that with doctoring, it's a very fine thing—any time you get an opportunity to keep the watch, and struggle with it, and come to know you did your best to help them prevail. . . .

Julia's Mother

Which brings me back, it seems, to where I began—to the tragic case of Julia. The young girl in the white dress who was killed in the car accident on her way to school last autumn.

I'd thought about the case often, afterward; replayed the resuscitation in my mind from time to time—the panic in that room with the stark white lights, hands reaching in to help, all the spilled blood, the acquiescing . . . then the dilemma of the aftermath, when I had to go to the Quiet Room to tell her mother. . . .

Each time I reconsidered the case, I felt sure we had done everything possible for her, had followed protocol. Yet I always had misgivings about it—as if, in some important way, the case was still open, raw, unfinished. *Why?* I've had deaths on my watch before—you never forget, you remember them all. But you go on, even if it's a child lost, and eventually move past the futility, move on to help others. Because after doing all you can for someone, even if it fails, you come to perceive that there are others waiting. Having to get on to take care of the others always got you moving again.

After doing all you can . . . used to be simpler to define. Not now, not for me. Because something changes in the middle part of life—once you realize that as much time has passed as there is to come. It makes you consider things differently. You get moody, pondering the vulnerability of trees. Used to be the seizure case was a success if I got the difficult IV in, gave the right medication, and stopped the seizure; now it seems the seizure case is only a success if I get the difficult IV in, give the right medication, stop the seizure—and cause the least amount of pain.

Seemed I couldn't shake the almost guilty feeling inside—to recall the raw pain that came out of Julia's mother, the helpless misery after I told her about her daughter's death. To have seen her life so frighteningly transformed, diminished to a meagerness—because of something I had to say—or was it because of something I had *failed* to say? Is "I'm sorry, she did not make it" ever enough to give to a parent afterward? No man can unfold the petals of a rose. But what else is there, after you've manipulated the science all you can—to no avail?

OCTOBER 15, 1999
THE EMERGENCY ROOM
CHILDREN'S HOSPITAL

It was some months after the case that I retrieved a phone-mail message at work. From a female caller. Her voice was low and indistinct, which caused me to miss her name.

"This is _____. Can you please call me back? I have some

questions about my daughter. My telephone number is. . . ."

Probably a routine request for a prescription refill, I thought as I dialed.

"Hello?" answered the same female voice on the other end.

"This is the doctor from Children's Hospital. I got a message asking me to call this number. I'm sorry, but I couldn't make out the name on the tape. Was it you?"

"Yes. Thank you for returning my call. This is Julia's mother. Do you remember me?"

I didn't. *Julia's mother?* This is a common predicament for an ER doctor. Parents see me out in public, come up to me at the mall or a grocery store or restaurant—and ask if I remember them. Most don't seem to realize I treat hundreds of patients each year. It's usually a single quick encounter, a blur, which makes it almost impossible to recall. Most times an ear infection is just an ear and an infection and another prescription for antibiotics. And yet to a parent their child going to the ER must seem like an unforgettable experience for all involved.

I thought hard on it for another uncomfortable moment—yet it was still unclear; I couldn't specifically recall a patient named Julia, or her mother. . . . And then it moved unceasingly through me—that inevitable succession of mental images: *Quiet Room, arms crossed, the pleading, torrents on that passing face, swooning low to the floor, sobbing. Julia's mother.* You never forget the deaths.

I felt a queer surge, from inside out—an intense flush of—of guilt.

"Why—yes, I do remember you."

"Weren't you the doctor in the ER the day my daughter Julia died?"

"Yes."

"Well, I'm calling to see if—if I could possibly ask you a few questions."

I didn't know what to expect. Could she be angry with me? Yet her voice sounded tentative. Did she want clarification on some technical medical issue about the case? A copy of the coroner's report? I couldn't recall being in a situation quite like this before—

"Of course. Go ahead."

"I don't know if you still remember the day of the accident, since it was a year ago. Exactly a year ago."

"I remember it very well."

She cleared her throat a bit. Then recounted some of the details from that morning—of the police coming to her house to tell of the accident; of her arriving at the hospital after Julia, and having to wait alone in the Quiet Room down the hall for some word; of my opening the door—and how she knew what I was going to say, just by looking at me—

"Even though it's been a year since the accident, it feels like one long day that just won't end. I never know what to do with myself. I see her raincoat and yellow boots in the hallway. I watch the school bus go past our house in the afternoon, and keep waiting for her to run around the corner, to come to me. Sometimes, when I wake in the middle of the night, the house is so dark and quiet—like a tomb—the clock just won't move;

there is nothing, for hours—*except the same question in my mind, over and over. . . .*"

There was a long, tense pause between us. I couldn't tell if she wanted me to speak to this. If she did, well, I didn't know what to say—

"I know I can't go back," she said. "But it's important that she knew I was there then. I can't bear the thought of her being alone at the end, hurt and scared like that, without her mother. . . . So, what I want to ask you is—can you tell me, Doctor, since you were with her at the end—can you say—*did I get there in time, before her soul went to heaven?*"

I knew what she was after. My reply was pure, almost automatic—"There's no question you got here in time. No question. She did not go without you—I'm sure of it."

My response seemed to come from outside of me, far beyond the limits of my thinking brain. No need for deliberate consideration. As if I'd been holding the answer all along.

After another pause, she asked, "How do you know?"

And in the next instant, it seemed as if each tragic case I'd ever managed was flashed across my consciousness, and I perceived the essence which united them—

"It's something I've experienced before, each time I've been with a parent who just lost a child. Something powerful takes over, after we do all we can and it fails. Call it what you will; to me, it's the power of the only unbreakable bond there is in this life. The only sure thing we ever have. And it's absolute between a mother and child. I've felt it so many times before, with each tragic case. And I felt the full force of it between you and Julia in the ER that day."

These words seemed to emit spontaneously from somewhere else. Even though I recognized the sentiment they expressed as being my own; and the reality they depicted as being inevitable, backed by the raw force of truth—

And yet I couldn't tell if it was enough, if it might give her something to hold on to; because she seemed to drift away. She spoke of her daughter, recounted the private monument of their life together. . . . "A mother never forgets the sound of her baby's cry," she said. I listened, let her carry the clock. Then, after what felt like a final pause in the conversation, I wished her good luck.

"Thank you for taking time with me," she said. "I have to go now, I can't talk anymore. *Please remember us. . . .*"

Please remember us. . . . I heard it echo as I hung up the phone. It wore a tract in my mind. . . .

Courage to bring a life forward into the world. Sometimes an epiphany; sometimes straining at particles of light in the midst of a great darkness. Loved a child—gave it movement, taught it language. Lost a child—and in the wake are hushed graveclothes on a narrow bed, a coagulate damming up your heart. Lost in whispers. Surely we were not created for this kind of suffering . . . yet the orange glow fades beyond the trees. . . .

• • •

It was some months later that I received this letter in the mail:

Dear Doctor:

Thank you for our conversation this past autumn. It was certainly helpful to share my grief with one who has experienced the sufferings of those with a similar loss.

It goes without saying that this has been a very difficult time for me. Everything just went numb inside for so long after the accident. Julia was my only child, you know. She was so beautiful, so lovely in her form and manner. And when she passed, it seemed the light was out of my life forever.

Then I began to have feelings again—strong feelings, urging me to have another child. But I couldn't bring myself to consider it after the tragedy—I was so afraid to try again, when it seemed there were no rules under heaven, no protection for the innocents. I kept wondering the same thing—Why did God allow this to happen?

How can you get on in life when there is no answer to satisfy that question?

Our talk made me realize something important—that even after the tragedy, the physical separation, you never lose contact with your child. They are yours, always. Julia is still very much with me, every day; she's the last thing on my mind at night before I sleep, the first thing each morning. Sometimes I can feel her moving inside me—like before, but in a different way. It doesn't scare me anymore. Her presence, and the love I will always feel for her, is still the most powerful blessing I've ever received in my life.

I want to feel it again. God willing, I know the love I'd

share with another baby can only enhance the love I feel for Julia, enhance my memory of her.

Thank you, for helping me put into words what I already understood in my heart.

As Always—
Julia's Mother

• • •

I didn't hear again from Julia's mother. So I don't know how her life turned out. I don't know if she ever did bring another child into the world after her daughter's death. Much less whether she found even a moment of quiet patience amidst the howling din of despair that seemed to drown out the music of her mortality.

And though I wondered about it all from time to time, I didn't feel the need to call her to find out. Because something important was clarified between us the last time we spoke; and I was sure I had done my best for her. Used all my knowledge and experience—everything reaped from passing through the many hallways, doors and quiet rooms—was integrated in a moment of certainty to help answer her question. Pushed the doctoring far beyond the scope of science and numbers and medical protocols; extended the compass, with a mystique that gets at the healing after science has done all it can—and fails. It was a culmination, of all the difficult and uncertain steps taken before—the culmination of a journey to understanding what it takes to become a truly finished doctor, a healer.

A life is like a line of linear white light moving across a silent grid. When a tragedy of misfortune intersects it, the luminosity is dispersed, and its course and clarity are altered forever. What I learned is that sometimes the doctoring interposes a prism—which is all that I did for Julia's mother—and it helps to order the scatter, to more clearly show the components for what they are.

Later that night I walked the cold streets alone, in private with my hood up. I felt older—but in a good way—because I could look back on what had happened, and know that something very important was finished; something between me and Julia's mother. And it felt good, to have been part of the workings of a single significant day in this life—to have had the opportunity to keep the watch. And, after struggling with it, to know that I'd done my best to help them prevail.